Food Pharmacies : A Guide to Nutraceutical Riches

Dr. Khushbu Gurjar
Ms. Anushree R K

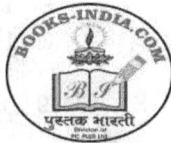

Pustak Bharati
Toronto Canada

Book Title : Food Pharmacies : A Guide to Nutraceutical Riches

Author : Dr. Khushbu Gurjar
　　　　　 Ms. Anushree R K

Published by :
Pustak Bharati (Books-India)
180 Torresdale Ave, Toronto Canada M2R 3E4
email : pustak.bharati.canada@gmail.com
Web : www.pustak-bharati-canada.com

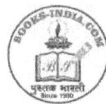

Copyright ©2024

ISBN 978-1-989416-19-8

ISBN : 978-1-989416-19-8

9 781989 416198

Acknowledgments

Writing a book is a journey that involves the support, encouragement, and contributions of numerous individuals and institutions. I am deeply grateful to all those whose guidance, assistance, and inspiration have made this endeavor possible.

First and foremost, I extend my heartfelt appreciation to my family for their unwavering love, understanding, and patience throughout this writing process. Their constant support has been my pillar of strength.

I extend my gratitude to my mentors, whose wisdom and guidance have shaped my understanding and fueled my passion for this subject. Your insights and encouragement have been invaluable in shaping the direction of this book.

I would also like to express my appreciation to the researchers, scientists, and experts whose groundbreaking work forms the foundation of the knowledge shared within these pages. Your dedication to advancing our understanding of nutraceuticals has been instrumental in shaping this book.

My sincere thanks also go to the publishers, editors, and everyone involved in the publication process. Your expertise, professionalism, and commitment have been instrumental in bringing this book to fruition.

Lastly, I want to express gratitude to the readers. Your curiosity and interest in exploring the world of nutraceuticals have been the driving force behind this work. It is my sincere hope that this book provides valuable insights and inspires a deeper appreciation for the transformative power of food.

Thank you all for being part of this journey.

Warm regards,

Dr. Khushbu Gurjar
Ms. Anushree R K

Contents

Preface

Welcome to the captivating world of nutraceuticals derived from diverse food sources! In an era where health and wellness have become paramount, the significance of what we consume has never been more critical. This book delves into the fascinating realm of nutraceuticals, exploring the wealth of beneficial compounds found in various foods that contribute to our well-being.

The term "nutraceutical" merges the concepts of nutrition and pharmaceuticals, encapsulating the idea that certain foods contain bioactive compounds with potential health benefits beyond their basic nutritional value. From ancient remedies to modern scientific discoveries, the utilization of these compounds to promote health, prevent diseases, and augment overall wellness has garnered significant attention.In this comprehensive volume, we embark on an enriching journey through the intricate tapestry of nutraceuticals sourced from an array of foods. Each chapter unveils the remarkable properties and therapeutic potential of these natural wonders, shedding light on their biochemical composition, physiological effects, and practical applications in promoting health.

From the polyphenols abundant in colorful fruits and vegetables to the omega-3 fatty acids found in oily fish, and from the antioxidant-rich spices to the medicinal herbs brimming with phytochemicals, this book meticulously explores the diverse classes of nutraceuticals available in nature's pantry. We unravel the mysteries behind these compounds, decipher their mechanisms of action, and elucidate how they positively impact human health. Moreover, as we navigate through these pages, we strive to bridge the gap between scientific research and practical implementation. While highlighting the potential health benefits, we also aim to provide insights into incorporating these nutraceuticals into daily diets, offering guidance on making informed choices for a healthier lifestyle.

This compilation is a testament to the collaborative efforts of experts in the fields of nutrition, biochemistry, pharmacology, and culinary arts. Their collective wisdom and dedication have culminated in this book, intended not only for scholars, researchers, and healthcare professionals but also for individuals eager to enhance their well-being through the power of food.As the world continues to recognize the pivotal role of nutrition in maintaining optimal health, this book serves as a beacon, illuminating the path toward harnessing the potential of nutraceuticals from diverse food sources. I sincerely hope this exploration into the realm of nutraceuticals enriches your understanding and empowers you to make informed choices for a healthier, more vibrant life.

With anticipation and excitement for the journey ahead,

Dr. Khushbu Gurjar
Ms. Anushree R K

Chapter -1

Introduction to Nutraceuticals

Introduction

Over the past few years, an increasing number of dietary supplements have become available in supermarkets and health food shops and even also available for purchase in pharmaceutical shops. The term "nutraceutical" is used to define these nutritionally or medicinally functional foods. Nutraceuticals, which have also been called medical foods, designer foods, functional foods, phytochemicals and nutritional supplements, comprise such everyday products as "bio" yoghurts and fortified breakfast cereals, as well as vitamins, herbal remedies and even genetically/living modified foods and supplements.

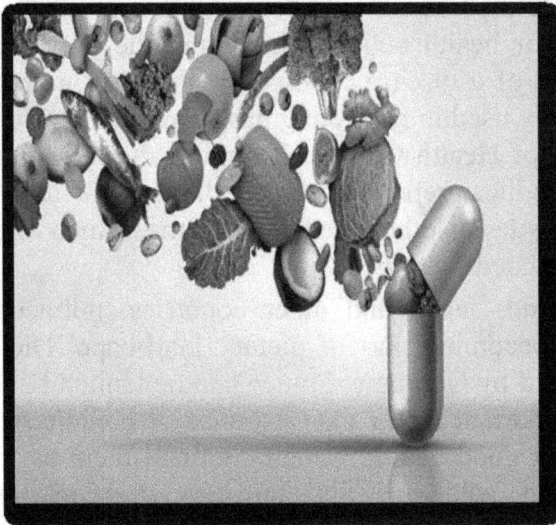

Many different terms and meanings are used in different countries, which can result in confusion. Nutraceuticals is a comprehensive umbrella term that is used to define any product resulting from food sources with extra health benefits in addition to the basic nutritional value found in foods. They can be considered non-specific biological therapies used to promote general well-being, prevent malignant processes and control symptoms. Generally, nutraceutical is said to be a "food, or parts of a food, that provide health benefits, including the prevention and treatment of disease.

History

The nutraceutical concept began from a survey conducted in the United Kingdom, Germany, and France, which concluded that consumers gave more importance to diet than to hereditary factors or to exercise to achieve good health. The term "nutraceutical" was coined from "nutrition" and "pharmaceutical" in 1989 by Stephen DeFelice, MD, founder and chairman of the Foundation for Innovation in Medicine (FIM), Cranford, NJ.1 According to DeFelice, nutraceutical can be defined as, "a food (or part of a food) that provides medical or health benefits, including the prevention and/or treatment of a disease." However, the term nutraceutical as commonly used in marketing has no regulatory definition. In the case of Health Canada, it defines the term nutraceutical as "a product prepared from food, but sold in the form of pills, powder or other medicinal forms, which are generally not associated with food"

In England, Japan and other countries, nutraceuticals are already becoming part of dietary landscape. Diet was first considered by Germany, France andthe United Kingdom as a more important factor than exercise or hereditary factors in achieving good health. Canada defined them as 'product of foods but sold in pills, powders, (potions) and other medicinal forms not normally associated with food'. In India, nutraceuticals are seen as the food components made from herbal or botanical raw materials, which are used for preventing or treating different types of chronic and acute maladies . Nowadays, nutraceuticals are one of the most rapidly growing segments of the industry with an expected

2

compound annual growth rate (CAGR) of 7.5% . The global nutraceutical market is estimated to increase from $241 billion market in 2019 to $373 billion in 2025 (Healthcare Packaging 2019). The definite use of nutraceuticals has been to achieve desirable therapeutic outcomes with reduced side effects. Herbal Nutraceuticals are powerful instruments in sustaining health and act contrary to nutritionally induced acute and chronic diseases by promoting optimal health, longevity and quality of life.

Scope

The philosophy behind nutraceuticals is focused on prevention. Most times it can be used in the context of Dietary supplements and/or functional food.

(a) Dietary Supplements: Dietary supplements are products envisioned to complement the diet that accepts or contains one or more of the following dietary ingredients: a mineral, a vitamin, an amino acid, a herb or other botanical, constituent, metabolite, a dietary substance for use by man to supplement the diet by increasing the total daily intake, or a concentrate, extract, or combinations of these ingredients. Dietary supplements are not intended to treat or remedy disease whereas nutraceuticals emphasize more on the expected results of these products, such as prevention or treatment of diseases.

(b) Functional Food: As defined by the United States of America Institute of Medicine's Food and Nutrition Board, functional food is "any food or food ingredient that may offer a health benefit beyond the traditional nutrients it contains". The functional food concept is – "Food products to be taken as part of the usual diet in order to have helpful effects that go beyond basic nutritional function". Functional foods contain physiologically active components obtained either from plants or animal sources .

Classification Nutraceuticals or functional foods can be classified on the basis of their sources:

Natural or traditional and Unnatural or non-traditional

(a) On the basis of natural source, it can be classified as the products obtained from plants, animals, minerals, or microbial sources. This classification can be referred to as Traditional Nutraceuticals.

(b) Nutraceuticals as prepared via biotechnology: this classification can be referred to as Non-Traditional Nutraceuticals.

Traditional Nutraceuticals

They are natural products with no changes to the food. They contain numerous natural components that convey benefits beyond basic nutrition, like omega-3 fatty acids in salmon, saponins in soy or lycopene in tomatoes. The traditional nutraceuticals can be divided on the basis of:

(a) Chemical Constituents. (i) Nutrients. (ii) Herbals. (iii) Phytochemicals.

(b) Nutraceutical Enzymes. (i) Chemical Constituents.

(c) Probiotic Microorganisms.

Nutrients

The nutrients include amino acids, fatty acids, minerals and vitamins with recognized nutritional functions. Most foods contain vitamins that aid in curing diseases like stroke, cataracts, osteoporosis and heart diseases. Minerals found in plants, animals and dairy products are useful in osteoporosis, anemia and in building strong bones, teeth, muscles, and improve nerve impulses and heart rhythm. Foods that contain fatty acids like omega-3 PUFAs are potent regulators of the inflammatory processes, maintenance of brain function and reduction in cholesterol deposition.

Herbals

Herbal nutraceuticals help to improve health and avert

4

chronic diseases. Most of these are analgesic, anti-inflammatory, astringent, antipyretic and antiarthritic. Some of the herbals contain flavonoids like apiol, psoralen that are diuretic, carminative and antipyretic. Peppermint (Menthapiperita) contains menthol as an active component that help cure cold and flu (Ehrlich 2009). Some of the plants contain tannin which is claimed to aid in the management of depression, cold, stress, cough, hypertension and asthma while proanthocyanadin found in some herbals are useful in the treatment or prevention of cancer, ulcers and urinary tract infections.

Phytochemicals
Phytochemicals are plant nutrients with particular biological activities that promote human health. They are also referred to as Phytonutrients. They work by serving as substrate for biochemical reactions, cofactors or inhibitors of enzymatic reactions, absorbents that bind to and eradicate unwanted constituent in the intestine and improve the absorption and/or stability of indispensable nutrients among others .

Nutraceutical Enzymes
These are enzymes that are derived from plant, animal and microbial sources. Enzymes are an essential part of life, without which our bodies would cease to function optimally. Medical conditions such as blood sugar disorders, digestive problems and obesity have their symptoms eliminated by enzyme supplements in the diet.

Probiotic Microorganisms
Probiotics mean 'for life'. They are defined as live microorganisms, which when consumed in tolerable amounts, confer a health effect on the host. These microorganisms are responsive bacteria that promote healthy digestion and absorption of some nutrients. They most importantly act to mob out pathogens, like yeasts and other bacteria and viruses that may cause disease and develop a

communally advantageous symbiosis with the human gastrointestinal tract. They possess an antimicrobial effect through altering the microflora, averting adhesion of pathogens to the intestinal epithelium, competing for nutrients necessary for pathogen survival, producing an antitoxin effect and retrogressing some of the consequences of infection on the intestinal epithelium, such as secretory changes and neutrophil migration. For instance, probiotics can cure lactose intolerance by enhancing the production of a specific enzyme (ß-galactosidase) that can hydrolyze the offending lactose into its component sugars.

Non-Traditional Nutraceuticals

These are the artificial foods developed via biotechnology. The bioactive components in food samples are engineered to produce products for human-wellness. They can be grouped into fortified nutraceuticals and recombinant nutraceuticals.

Fortified Nutraceuticals :

These are nutraceuticals from agrarian breeding or added nutrients and/or ingredients. Examples include cereals with added vitamins or minerals, milk fortified with cholecalciferol used in vitamin D deficiency, flour with added folic acid, prebiotic and probiotic fortified milk with Bifidobacteriumlactis HN019 used in diarrhea, respiratory infections and severe illnesses, in children , and orange juice fortified with calcium.

Recombinant Nutraceuticals :

Recombinant nutraceuticals include the making of probiotics and the extraction of bioactive components by enzyme/fermentation technologies as well as genetic engineering technology. Also, energy-providing foods, such as bread, alcohol, fermented starch, yoghurt, cheese, vinegar, and others are produced using modern biotechnology. Examples include cows with lactoferrin deficiency is engineered with recombinant human lactoferrin (rhLf) to be able to solve the lactoferrin deficiency.

Examples of functional foods/ nutraceuticals their source and uses

S. No.	Functional Ingredients	Source	Medicinal use
1	Carotenoids:- Alpha-Carotenoids Beta-Carotenoids	Carrots, Fruits Vegetables	Neutralize free radicals may cause damage to cells
2	Lutein	Green vegetables	Reduce the risk of muscular degeneration
3	Lycopene	Tomato products (ketch up, sauces)	Reduce the risk of prostate cancer.
4	Dietary fibre Insoluble fibre	Wheat, bran	Reduce the risk of breast or colon cancer.
5	Beta glucan Soluble fibre	Oats, barley, psyllium	Reduce the risk of cardiovascular disease. Protect against heart disease and some cancers, lower LDL and total cholesterol.
6	Fatty acids:- Long chain omega- 3 fatty acid DHA/EPA	Salmon and other fish oil	Reduce the risk of cardiovascular diseases, improve mental, visual functions.
7	Conjugated linoleic	Cheese, meat products	Improve body composition,

			decrease risk of certain cancers.
	acid(CLA)		
8	Phenolics:- Anthracyanides Catechins Flavonones Lignans	Fruits, Tea, Citrus, vegetables Flax, rye	Neutralize free radicals, reduce the risk of cancer of stomach and oesophagus. Prevention of cancer, renal failure
9	Tannins (proanthocyanidines)	Cranberries, cranberry products, coca, chocolate	Improve urinary tract , reduce risk of cardiovascular diseases.
10	Plant sterols:- Stanol ester	Corn, soy, wheat, wood oil	Lower blood cholesterol levels by inhibiting cholesterol absorption.
11	Prebiotics/ Probiotics:- Fructo-oligosaccharides	Jerusalem artichokes, shallots, onion powder	Improve quality of intestinal microflora,gastrointestinal health
12	Lactobacillus	Yogurt, other dairy products	
13	Soya phytoestrogens:- Isoflavones, Daidzein, Genistein	Soyabeans and soy based foods	Menopause symptoms such as hot flashes. Protect against heart disease and some cancers, lowers LDL and total cholesterol.

Market trends of nutraceuticals

The nutraceutical industry's three main segments include functional foods, dietary supplements, and herbal/natural products. Nutrition Business Journal (NBJ) identified an $80 billion nutraceuticals market in 1995 by considering natural and organic foods ($6.2 billion), functional foods ($13.4 billion), certain lesser-evil foods with reduced or no unhealthy ingredients ($23 billion), dietary supplements ($8.9 billion), and selected market standard foods ($28.3 billion). NBJ has begun tracking nutraceuticals industry growth. Since 1995, the industry, as defined by NBJ, has grown by an average of 7.1 percent per year. In 1997, industry sales totaled $91.7 billion (NBJ 1998). The most rapidly growing segments of the industry were dietary supplements (19.5 percent per year) and natural/herbal products (11.6 percent per year) . According to BCC Research - The global nutraceuticals market grew to $46.7 billion in 2002, at an AAGR of nearly 7%. In 2007 nutraceuticals sale is projected to reach $74.7 billion at an AAGR of 9.9%. This assumes a world economic recovery in 2003 and an end to price competition.

The future of nutraceuticals

Increasing awareness levels about fitness and health, spurred by media coverage are prompting the majority of people to lead healthier lifestyles, exercise more, and eat healthy. The expanding nutraceutical market indicates that end users are seeking minimally processed food with extra nutritional benefits and organoleptic value. This development, in turn, is propelling expansion in the nutraceutical markets globally. The emerging nutraceuticals industry seems destined to occupy the landscape in the new millennium. Its tremendous growth has implications for the food, pharmaceutical, healthcare, and agricultural industries Many scientists believe that enzymes represent another exciting frontier in nutraceuticals. "Enzymes have been underemployed... they're

9

going to be a hot area in the future." Fermentation technology using microbes to create new food products also represents potential. Global trends to healthy products cannot be reversed. Companies taking the lead by investing strategically in science, product development, marketing and consumer education will not go unrewarded.

Conclusion

The nutraceutical industry is growing at a rate far exceeding expansion in the food and pharmaceutical industries. In tomorrow's market, the most successful nutraceutical players are likely to be those companies in which functional product are just a part of a broad line of goods satisfying both conventional and health value point. Future demand of nutraceutical depends on consumer perception of the relationship between diet and disease. Although nutraceuticals have significant promise in the promotion of human health and disease prevention ,health professional, nutritionists and regulatory toxicologist should strategically work together to plan appropriate regulation to provide the ultimate health and therapeutic benefit to mankind. Long-term clinical studies are required to scientifically validate the nutraceuticals in various medical conditions. The interaction of nutraceuticals with food and drugs is another area, which should be taken into consideration. The effect of different processing methods on the biological availability and effectiveness of nutraceuticals remains to be determined. As like drugs, there should be strict regulatory controls for nutraceuticals.

References

1. Chauhan B, Kumar G, Kalam N, Ansari SH (2013) Current concepts and prospects of herbal nutraceutical: a review. J Adv Pharm Technol Res 4(1):4–8

2. Ernst E (2001) Functional foods, nutraceuticals, designer foods: innocent fad or counterproductive marketing ploy. Eur J Clin Pharmacol 57:353–355
3. Healthcare Packaging (2019) The global market for nutraceuticals set for robust growth. Available: https://www.healthcarepackaging.com/markets/neutraceut icals-functional/article/13296428/ the-global-market-for-nutraceuticals-set-for-robust-growth. Retrieved 6th January 2020
4. Holzapfel WH, Haberer P, Geisen R, Bjorkroth J, Schillinger U (2001) Taxonomy and important features of probiotic microorganisms in food and nutrition. Am J Clin Nutr 73:365S–373S
5. Hyvonen P, Suojala L, Orro T, Haaranen J, Simola O, Rontved C, Pyorala SP (2006) Transgenic cows that produce recombinant human lactoferrin in milk are not protected from experimental Escherichia coli Intramammary Infection. Infect Immun 74:6206–6212
6. Kalra, E. K. (2003). Nutraceutical-definition and introduction. *Aaps Pharmsci*, *5*(3), 27-28.
7. Michail S, Sylvester F, Fuchs G, Issenma R (2006) Clinical efficacy of probiotics: Review of the evidence with focus on children, clinical practice guideline. J Pediatr Gastroenterol Nutr 43(4)
8. Nutrition Business Journal, 1:2, September 1996
9. Oak SJ, Jha R (2019) The effects of probiotics in lactose intolerance: A systematic review. Crit Rev Food Sci Nutr 59(11):1675–1683
10. Pandey, M., Verma, R. K., & Saraf, S. A. (2010). Nutraceuticals: new era of medicine and health. *Asian J Pharm Clin Res*, *3*(1), 11-15.
11. Rishi RK. Nutraceutical: borderline between food and drug. Pharma Review 2006, Available from: http://www.kppub.com/articles/herbal-safety-

pharmareview-004/nutraceuticals-borderline-between-food-anddrugs.html. Accessed on date Feb 12, 2009.
12. Sazawal S, Dhingra U, Hiremath G, Sarkar A, Dhingra P, Dutta A, Verma P, Menon VP, Black RE (2010) Prebiotic and probiotic fortified milk in prevention of morbidities among children: community-based, randomized, double-blind, controlled trial. PLoS One 5:e12164
13. Thakur N, Gupta BP, Nagariya AK, Jain NP, Banweer J, Jain S (2010) Nutraceutical: New Era's safe pharmaceuticals. J Pharm Res 3:1243–1247
14. Zeisel SH (1999) Regulation of "Nutraceuticals". Science 285:185–186
15. Zhao J (2007) Nutraceuticals, nutritional therapy, phytonutrients, and phytotherapy for improvement of human health: a perspective on plant biotechnology application. Bentham Science Publishers. Available from: http://www.benthamscience.com/biot/samples/biot1-1/Zhao.pdf. Last accessed 03 April, 2019

Chapter -2

Garlic and its Health Benefits

Introduction

Garlic is a natural health promoter and a miracle drug available in the lap of nature.. Botanically it is known as Allium sativum and is a member of the Alliaceae or Family Liliaceae . Due to its strong odorous nature, garlic it is commonly known as stinking rose. Garlic is the oldest cultivated grass. Its origin is linked to Central Asia. The Sumerians were the first to use it as a medicine. The individual part of garlic is known as garlic clove. Allicin is the active component of garlic. It is formed by crushing or cutting the garlic clove. Allicin gives garlic its pungency along with a large amount of health benefits. It is a rich in protein, calcium, magnesium, iron, potassium, zinc, arginine, saponins, polyphenols and selenium. It's also filling source of some vitamins such as vitamin A, vitamin B6 and B1 and vitamin C. Garlic is commonly used as a spice and seasoning in the various cuisines of the world.

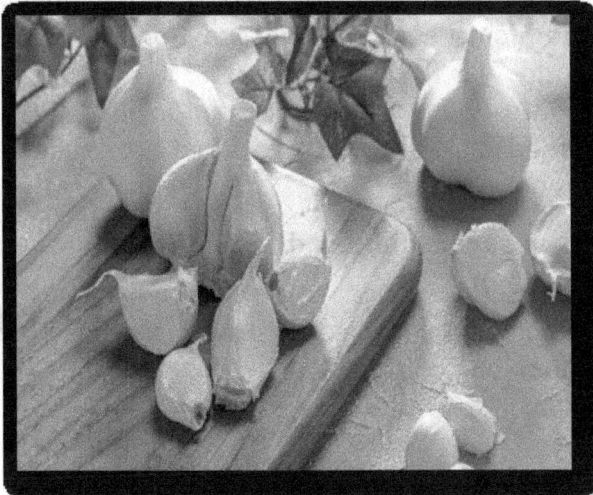

Geographical and agronomic features about Garlic

It's a indispensable ingredient in Asian, French and Italian cuisine cooking. In general, it is classified into two main ones categories: hard neck and soft neck. Garlic is a small underground bulb crop .In India Garlic is grown in the low lands during the months of October to March. In the northern hills it is grown from September to June and in southern hills from May to October. It mainly grown with vegetative propagation.

History about garlic

The letter garlic comes from the Old English word garleac i.e. throwing the leek. The 'gar' means spear (referring to the spear shaped leaves) and "leac" means leek. The origin of garlic dates back to 5,000-6,000 years ago, it is originally from Central Asia. But it is difficult to trace the country of origin. During the 18th century in France undertakers crush whole garlic into wine. they had a strong belief that by consuming this preparation, they would protect themselves from the deadly disease called to plague. In 1722, garlic was the main ingredient of "The vinegar of the four thieves", adapted to protect against the plague. Soldiers in World War I and World War II were given garlic to prevent gangrene1. It was also used as an antiseptic and applied to wounds to prevent infection. Garlic was even used as currency due to its high rates during this era.

Varieties of garlic found in different regions

Garlic varieties have been renowned many times like them passed among farmers and gardeners. Garlic is descended from Allium longicus pis.

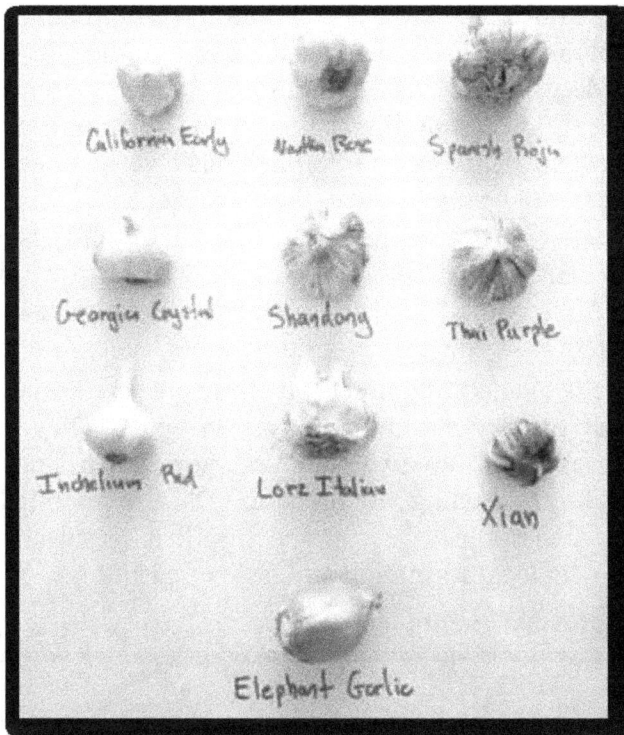

California Early   Nadda Rose   Spanish Roja

Georgian Crystal   Shandong   Thai Purple

Inchelium Red   Lorz Italian   Xian

Elephant Garlic

- The "wild garlic", "crow garlic", e "field garlic" of Great Britain are members of the Allium species ursinum, Allium vineale and Allium oleraceum, respectively.
- In North America, Allium vineale and Allium canadense (meadow garlic/wild onion) are common weeds found in fields and Elephant garlic is one of the best known garlics (Allium ampeloprasus).
- Single Garlic Clove (Pearl/Single Garlic) originally from the Chinese province of Yunnan. a lot of garlic cultivars have names indicating where they were found traditionally farmed or the color of their coat, inclusive 'Oregon Blue', 'Chinese Pink', 'Chesnok Red' and 'Spanish Red'.
- They are American garlic, Mexican garlic and Italian garlic the top 3 varieties available in the US The

young/immature garlic with a long green top and a white bulb it is known as green garlic. Raven garlic (A. vineale) is widely spread and common in many districts. their bulbs are very small. Ramsons (A. ursinum) grow in forests and it gives small bulbs. It has a very pungent taste and a strong smell. They they are generally known as 'broadleaf garlic'. Field Garlic (A. oleraceum) is a rare plant. There are many species of garlic grown in the garden. A. odorum and A. fragrans have fragrant flowers, but these have the aroma of garlic in its leaves and roots.

So garlic is available in numerous forms. These varieties are the result of random mutations of the past. They can be widely classified into two main categories: hard neck and soft neck. According to genetic DNA variability and weather conditions we can see significant impact on the garlic flower stem formation and taste of garlic.

Chemical constituents

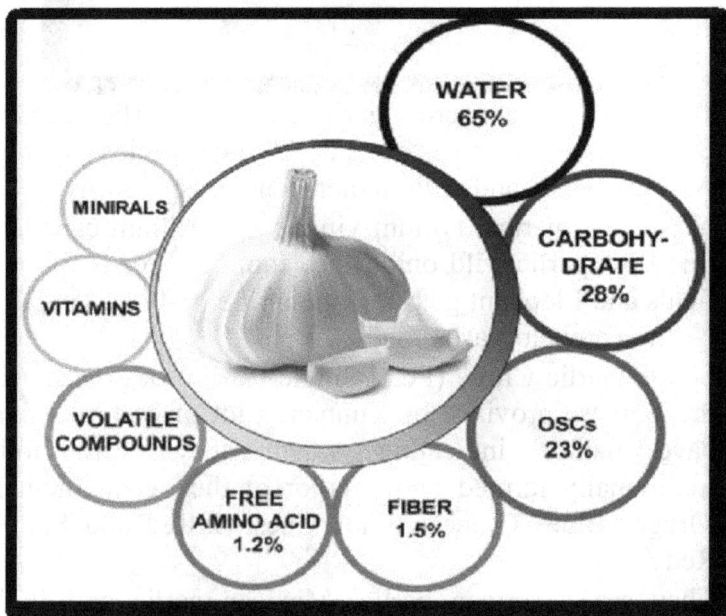

Garlic contains about 0.1% volatile oil and this oil is rich in sulfur content and devoid of oxygen. The main constituents of the oil are diallyl disulfide (60%), diallyl trisulfide (20%), allyl propyl disulfide (6%), a small amount of diethyl disulfide and probably diallyl polysulfide. These sulfur compounds contribute to both the smell and taste of garlic. The active properties of garlic are due to this spicy volatile oil.

The garlic bulb is made up of 84.09% water, 13.38% from organic matter and 1.53% inorganic matter. There are 20 kinds of sulfur compounds (eg, allicin, methyl allyl trisulfide e diallyl trisulfide) reported in garlic. Seven organosulfurs compounds such as Alliin, isoalliin, methiin, cycloalliin, e gamma-1-glutamyl-S-methyl-1-cysteine was also determined in it. Allicin is chemically and therapeutically active constituent of garlic. Allicin is released only by crushing or chews raw garlic and cannot be formed from cooked garlic. It is a colorless, odorless and water soluble component. The fermented garlic product had a higher content of riboflavin, α-tocopherol, but lower thiamin level compared to unfermented product. The macerated oil garlic contains iso-E-10-devinylajoene, Z-10-devinylajoene, and three or five thiosulfinates. vitamins (Vit-B1, B2, B3, B5, B6, B9 and C) proteins rich in arginine, mineral salts (calcium, iron, magnesium, manganese, phosphorus, potassium, sodium,zinc, selenium), saponins, oligosaccharides, dietary fibers and flavonoids.

Nutraceuticals health benefits of garlic

The nutraceutical property of garlic has so many health benefits . Some of the important health benefits are listed below and the pictorial representation is given in figure 1.

17

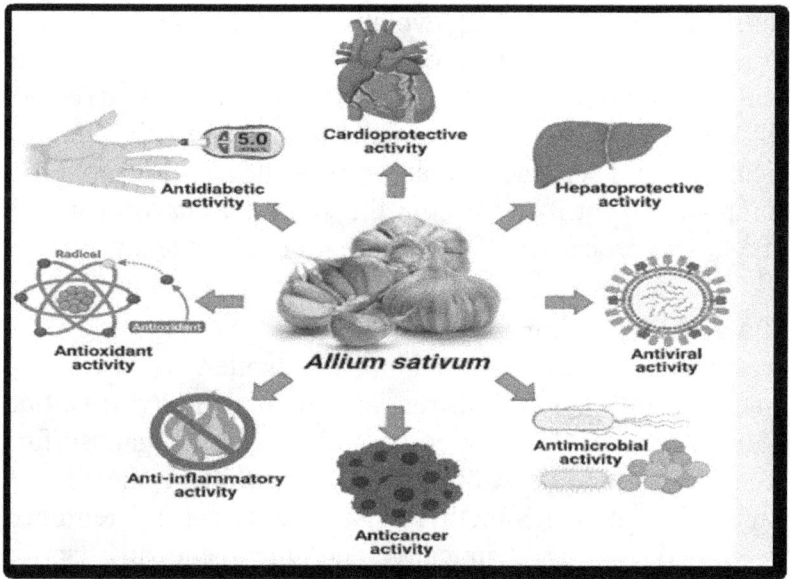

Fig 1: Health benefits of Garlic

I. Good for Heart

The positive effect of garlic on the circulatory system is very well documented. Several large studies have shown that taking supplements that mimic fresh garlic can significantly lower LDL cholesterol levels without harming beneficial HDL cholesterol levels. Garlic appears to work by preventing the liver from making too much LDL cholesterol. There is also some evidence that garlic supplements may lower blood pressure slightly by dilating or expanding blood vessels and garlic helps prevent blood clots and therefore reduces the risk of heart attack and stroke by decreasing the viscosity of platelets, which are tiny, disc-shaped bodies in the blood needed for blood to clot. When platelets are too sticky, they form lumps that can stick to artery walls and contribute to clogged arteries. It also stimulates the production of nitric oxide in the lining of blood vessel walls, a substance that helps them relax.

According to a study published in Life Sciences, a daily dose of 1 ml/kg of body weight of garlic extract over a period of 6 months resulted in a significant reduction of oxidative stress (free radicals) in the blood of patients suffering from arteriosclerosis. Its positive effect on the circulatory system improves blood flow throughout the body, which is why it has also been hailed as a cure for impotence

The medicinal health benefits of garlic include improved blood circulation. Garlic contains a certain chemical compound called allicin which is converted into another compound called ajoene. Ajoene works as an effective suppressant of blood clots or cholesterol in the human body, so it works as a blood thinner. Thus, it is extremely helpful in treating conditions like atherosclerosis and thrombosis, which are caused by the thickening of the blood. Garlic and Blood Clots Another medicinal health benefit of garlic is its effects on blood clots. Aioene, a compound made after garlic is crushed or minced, is said to be an anticoagulant substance that reduces the formation of blood clots. Studies from Saarland University in Germany have also shown that compounds in garlic help blood clots dissolve more quickly; they also improve blood flow. In India, 50 people who ate 3 cloves of raw garlic a day are said to have experienced improvements in blood clotting time and clot-dissolving activity of about 20%. Garlic and the immune system Not surprisingly, the presence of all these antioxidants in garlic has a very positive effect on the immune system in general and can therefore protect the body from all types of bacterial and viral attacks. Research has also recently shown that it has an inhibitory effect on MSRA, which is currently wreaking havoc in UK hospitals.

II. Cancer
Reduces the size of some cancerous tumors and helps prevent some types of cancer, especially those of the intestine. Garlic and Cancer Current research has shown that

a number of readily available foods, such as garlic and onions, that make up a healthy diet actually have a major impact on cancer prevention. The protective effect of garlic appears to be greater than that of onion, although onion consumption has been shown to reduce the risk of stomach cancer. These anticancer foods appear to have the ability to interfere with the development of cancerous tumors. The October 2000 issue of the American Journal of Nutrition reported a summary of a number of epidemiological studies showing that people who regularly ate cooked or raw garlic compared with those who ate little or no garlic had about half the risk of colorectal cancer. stomach and a third lower risk of colorectal cancer. This amazing little bulb is now at the top of the American National Cancer Institute's list of possible cancer-prevention foods. Contains multiple anti-cancer and antioxidant compounds, more than 30 at last count, powerful compounds such as quercetin, diallyl sulfide, allin and ajoene. These have the ability to block carcinogens such as nitrosamine and aflatoxins, which have been specifically linked to stomach, lung and liver cancer. The ajoene and allicin in garlic have also been shown to slow down cancer cells as a type of natural chemotherapy.The Iowa Women's Health Study found that women who included garlic in their daily diets had lower risks of colon cancer.

III. Antibiotic

However, one of the oldest uses of garlic is as an antibiotic. The fresh garlic kills a variety of microbes, including viruses, bacteria, fungi and parasites and can be effective against conditions such as athlete's foot, thrush (a fungal infection of the mouth), viral diarrhea and the bacteria Helicobacter pylori which causes ulcers. Available in pills, capsules, liquids, and raw cloves, garlic is one of the most popular health herbs today.

IV. Lungs function

a) Tuberculosis : Garlic is also useful in treating tuberculosis. In Ayurveda, a decoction of garlic boiled in milk is considered a miracle drug for tuberculosis.

b) Asthma : It should be taken three times a day. Taken in sufficient quantities, it is a wonderful remedy for pneumonia. Asthma: This has been found effective in reducing the severity of asthma attacks.

c) Cold and cough : Garlic also acts as a good cold medicine, decongestant and expectorant. Home Remedies Garlic is an invaluable remedy for asthma, hoarseness, cough, tonsillitis, shortness of breath and most other ailments of the lungs, being of particular virtue in chronic bronchitis owing to its power to promote expectoration. An old asthma remedy, which used to be the most popular, is a garlic syrup, made by boiling garlic bulbs until soft and adding an equal amount of vinegar to the water in which they were boiled, and then sweetened and boiled until a syrup is obtained. The syrup is then poured over the boiled garlic bulbs, which have in the meantime been dried, and stored in a jar. Every morning you should take a bulb or two, with a spoonful of syrup.

V. Antioxidant properties

The antioxidant properties of garlic help scavenge harmful free radicals, which can damage LDL (bad) cholesterol in the blood.

VI. Brain function

Studies on garlic and brain animals have shown improved brain function after eating garlic. It is possible that the antioxidants in garlic neutralize and destroy free radicals that accumulated in the body. Garlic useful in treating people with Alzheimer's disease, which is caused by the accumu-lation of free radicals. Researchers in China have also shown that the sulfur compound salicycysteine found in garlic prevents degeneration of the frontal lobes of the brain. Therefore, eating garlic can even make you smarter.

VII. Digestive Disorders

Garlic is one of the most important herbs for the digestive system. Stimulates peristalsis or bowel movement and the secretion of digestive juices.

VIII. Rheumatism/Arthritis

Garlic has also been shown to reduce pain and other symptoms in people with rheumatoid arthritis. In Russia, garlic is widely used in the treatment of rheumatism and associated diseases. Even in Britain, garlic is recommended for rheumatic conditions.

IX. Blood Disorders

The herb is considered to be a rejuvenator. It has been found to help eliminate toxins, revitalize the blood, stimulate circulation and promote intestinal flora or bacteria colonies which prevents infection by harmful bacteria.

X. Skin Disorders

Garlic has been used successfully for a variety of skin ailments. Pimples disappear without scars when rubbed with raw garlic several times a day. Even very persistent forms of acne in some adults have been cured with garlic. Garlic rubbed on ringworm provides quick relief. The area is burned by the strong garlic and then the skin peels off and the ringworm heals.

XI. Immune functioning

It's a surprisingly good source of vitamins C, B6, and the minerals selenium and manganese, which have long been associated with boosting the immune system, among other benefits.

XII. Garlic and weight management

Garlic Aids Weight Management Allicin is the most potent

substance in garlic and has been shown to not only lower blood pressure, insulin and triglyceride levels in laboratory animals fed a high sugar diet, but also prevent even weight gain. A study published in the American Journal of Hypertension reported that animals that developed high insulin levels, hypertension, and high triglycerides were either given allicin or served as a control. Although all animals consumed the same amount of food, weight only increased in the control group, while animals that were supplemented with allicin maintained a stable weight or even noticed a slight decrease. The researchers concluded that allicin may have practical value for weight control.

XIII. Other uses

Garlic has a pronounced aphrodisiac effect. It is a tonic for loss of potency for any reason. It also treats sexual weakness and impotence caused by excessive sex and nervous exhaustion from habit dissipation. It is said to be especially helpful for seniors with nervous tension and low libido and it also helpful for ear infections. Garlic can cure pain caused by insect bites such as scorpions and centipedes.

Recommended Daily Allowance for Garlic

There is no set recommended daily allowance for garlic. As with any herb or supplement, too much may not be beneficial and garlic is no exception. Eating too much garlic can irritate the digestive tract. A beneficial and safe amount for those who like fresh garlic is to eat 1-2 cloves a day. To avoid the dreaded garlic breath, you might choose your garlic in capsule form. If you prefer garlic capsules, the commonly suggested amount is 600-900 mg (providing approximately 5,000-6,000 mcg of allicin) divided into 2-3 equal amounts. When using aged garlic extracts, a suggested supplement is 3-7 grams per day.

Conclusion

In conclusion, garlic's nutraceutical properties hold

tremendous potential for various aspects of human health. Its long-standing reputation as a medicinal herb is being supported by scientific research, which continues to unveil the diverse range of benefits associated with garlic consumption. From its antimicrobial effects to cardiovascular health, anticancer properties, immune system support, neuroprotective effects, gut health modulation, and anti-inflammatory and antioxidant properties, garlic showcases a multifaceted arsenal of bioactive compounds.

While further investigation is required to fully comprehend the mechanisms behind these effects and optimize the development of garlic-based nutraceuticals, the future looks promising. The identification and isolation of specific garlic compounds responsible for its health benefits may lead to targeted interventions and the creation of more potent and standardized nutraceutical products.

It is important to emphasize that incorporating garlic or its derived nutraceuticals into one's routine should be done under the guidance of healthcare professionals, especially for individuals with specific health conditions or taking medications. Additionally, future research should explore potential synergistic effects of garlic with other natural compounds or pharmaceutical agents, as well as conduct rigorous clinical trials to validate its efficacy and safety profiles.

In conclusion, garlic's journey as a nutraceutical powerhouse continues to unfold, offering a rich source of possibilities for enhancing human health and well-being. As our understanding deepens and scientific advancements progress, garlic may hold the key to novel therapeutic approaches and improved health outcomes for individuals around the globe.

References

1. Haciseferogullari H, Ozcan M, Demir F, Calisir S. Some nutritional and technological properties of garlic (Allium sativum L.). J Food Eng 2005; 68: 463-69. http://dx.doi.org/10.1016/j.jfoodeng.2004.06.024
2. .Nagakubo T, Nagasawa A, Okhawa H. Micropropagation of garlic through in vitro bulblet formation. Plant Cell Tiss Org Cult 1993; 32(2): 175-83. http://dx.doi.org/10.1007/BF00029840 /1471-2261-8-13 7599.2003.tb00268.x
3. Alder R, Lookinland S, Berry JA, Williams M. A systematic review of the effectiveness of garlic as an anti-hyperlipidemic agent. J Am Acad Nurse Pract 2003; 15(3): 120-9. http://dx.doi.org/10.1111/j.1745-
4. Almogren A, Shakoor Z, Adam M. Garlic and onion sensitization among Saudi patients screened for food allergy: a hospital based study. Afr Health Sci 2013; 13(3): 689-93.
5. Amagase H, Petesch BL, Matsuura H, Kasuga S, Itakura Y. Intake of garlic and its bioactive components. J Nutr 2001: 131(3s): 955S-62S.
6. Bekheet AS. A synthetic seed method through encapsulation of in vitro proliferated bulblets of garlic (Allium sativum L.). Arab J Biotech 2006; 9(3): 415-26.
7. Borrelli F, Capasso R, Izzo AA. Garlic (Allium sativum L.): adverse effects and drug interactions in humans. Mol Nutr Food Res 2007; 51(11): 1386-97. http://dx.doi.org/10.1002/mnfr.200700072
8. Breithaupt-Grogler, K., et al. Circulation 96(8): 2649-2655, 1997.
9. Cardelle Cobas A, Soria AC, Corzo Martinez M, Villamiel M. A Comprehensive Survey of Garlic Functionality. In: Pãcurar M and Krejci G, editors. Garlic Consumption and Health. New York: Nova

10. Dillon SA, Burmi RS, Lowe GM, et al. Life Sci. 2003; 72(14): 1583-1594. doi.org/10.1007/s00122-004-1815-5
11. Dorant E, van den Brandt PA, Goldbohm RA, Hermus RJ, Sturmans F. Br J Cancer. 1993; 67(3): 424-429.
12. Dorant E, van den Brandt PA, Goldbohm RA. Breast Cancer Res Treat. 1995; 33(2): 163- 170.
13. Dorant E, van den Brandt PA, Goldbohm RA. Carcinogenesis. 1996; 17(3): 477-484.
14. Durak I, Kavutcu M, Aytaç B, Avci A, Devrim E, Ozbek H, Oztürk HS. Effects of garlic extract consumption on blood lipid and oxidant/antioxidant parameters in humans with high blood cholesterol. J
15. Fenwick GR, Hanley AB. The genus Allium- Part1. Crit Rev Food Sci Nutr 1985; 22(3): 199-271. http://dx.doi.org/10.1080/104083 98509527415
16. Fleischauer AT, Arab L. Garlic and cancer: a critical review of the epidemiologic literature. J Nutr 2001; 131: 1032S-1040S.
17. Gupta RP. Garlic cultivation technology. J Spices aromatic Crop 1998; 9(l): 1-8.
18. Herbs of the Bible: 2000 Years of Plant Medicine - James A. Duke, PhD. 1999, Interweave Press.
19. Ipek M, Ipek A, Almquist SG, Simon PW. Demonstration of linkage and development of the first low-density genetic map of garlic, based on AFLP markers Theor Appl Genet 2005; 110 (2): 228-236. http://dx.J 2003; 24(8): 842-45.
20. Kyo, E., et al. Phytomedicine 4(4): 335-340, 1997.
21. Lanzotti V. The analysis of onion and garlic. J Chromatogr A 2006; 1112 (1-2): 3-22. http://dx.doi.org/10.1016/j.chroma.2005.12.016
22. Maas HI, Klaas M. Intra specific differentiation of garlic (Alli um sativum L.) by isozyme and RAPD markers. Theor Appl Genet 1995; 91(1): 89-97. Nutr

Biochem 2004; 15(6): 373-7. http://dx.doi.org/10.1016/j.jnutbio.2004.01.005
23. Parle M, Kumar Vaibhav. Garlic-A Delicious Medicinal Nutrient. In: Trivedi PC, editor. Indian Folk Medicine. Jaipur, India: Pointer Publisher; 2007. p. 210-29.
24. Parle M, Kaura S. A hot way leading to healthy stay. Int Res J Pharm 2012; 3(6): 21-5.
25. Parle M, Kaura S. How to live with Rheumatoid Arthritis??? Int Res J Pharm 2012; 3(3): 115-21
26. Parle M, Kaura S, Sethi N, Jena P. Role of Media in safe guarding health of the society. Int Res J Pharm 2013; 4(10): 16-20. http://dx.doi.org /10.7897/2230-8407.041005
27. Parle M, Kaura S, Sethi N. Understanding Gout beyond Doubt. Int Res J Pharm 2013; 4(9): 25-34. http://dx.doi.org/10.7897/2230-8407.04907
28. Prescription for Nutritional Healing, Third Edition. James F. Balch, M.D., Phyllis A. Balch, C.N.C., Avery Publishing Group, 2000.
29. Ried K, Frank OR, Stocks NP, Fakler P, Sullivan T. Effect of garlic on blood pressure: a systematic review and meta- analysis. BMC Cardiovasc Disord 2008; 8: 13. http://dx.doi.org/10.1186
30. Ross SA, Finley JW, Milner JA. Allyl sulfur compounds from garlic modulate aberrant crypt formation. J Nutr 2006; 136(3 Suppl): 852S–4S.
31. Salih BA, Abasiyanik FM. Does regular garlic intake affect the prevalence of Helicobacter pylori in asymptomatic subjects? Saudi Med
32. Salih BA, Abasiyanik FM. Saudi Med J. 2003; 24(8): 842-845.
33. Sarrell EM, Mandelberg A, Cohen HA. Arch Pediatr Adolesc Med. 2001; 155: 796-799.

34. Sata SJ, Shagatharia SB, Thaker VS. Induction of direct somatic embryogenesis in garlic. Methods in Cell Sci 2000; 22(4): 299-304. http://dx.doi.org/10.1023/A:1017541500318
35. Scharbert G, Kalb ML, Duris M, Marschalek C, Kozek-Langenecker SA. Anesth Analg. 2007; 105(5): 1214-8. Science Publishers; 2010. p. 1-60.
36. Siegers CP, Steffen B, Robke A, Pentz R. Phytomedicine. 1999; 6(1): 7-11.
37. Silagy CA, Neil AW. J Hypertens. 1994; 12: 463-468.
38. Spigelski D, Jones PJ. Nutr Rev. 2001; 59(7): 236-241.
39. Steiner M, Khan AH, Holbert D, Lin RI. Am J Clin Nutr. 1996; 64: 866–870.
40. Steinmetz KA, Kushi LH, Bostick RM, Folsom AR, Potter JD. Am J Epidemiol. 1994; 139(1): 1-15.
41. Stevinson C, Pittler MH, Ernst E. Ann Intern Med. 2000; 133(6): 420-429.
42. Superko HR, Krauss RM. J Am Coll Cardiol. 2000; 35(2): 321-326.
43. Sushma K, Manju S, Grewal S, Koul S, Sambyal M. Embryogenesis and plantlet formation in garlic (Allium sativum L.). J Spices aromatic 1994; 3(1): 43 -7.
44. The Encyclopedia of Medicinal Plants - Andrew Chevalier, 1996 DK Publishing, London.
45. The Green Pharmacy - James A. Duke, PhD. 1997 Rodale Press.
46. The Herbal Encyclopedia - A Practical Guide to the Many Uses of Herbs by Rev. Dr. Lisa Waltz, 1999-2000. www.earthnow.org.
47. The Herbalist, newsletter of the Botanic Medicine Society. December 1988.
48. Tripathi PC, Lawande KE. Effect of gamma rays irradiation on storage behavior in garlic (Allium sativum L.) J Spices aromatic Crop 2006; 16(1): 22–6.

49. Volk GM, Henk AD, Richards CM. Genetic Diversity among U.S. Garlic Clones a s Detected Using AFLP Methods. J Amer Soc Hort Sci 2004; 129(4): 559-69.
50. Walkey D, Webb MJW, Bolland CJ, Miller A. Production of virus-free garlic (Allium sativum L.) and shallot (A. ascalonicum L.) by meristem-tip culture. J Hortic Sci Biotech 1987; 62(2): 211–20.

Chapter-3

Health benefits of Omega 3 Fatty Acids

Introduction

Omega-3 fatty acids, also known as omega-3s, are vital polyunsaturated fats crucial for the maintenance of a healthy body. Since our bodies are incapable of producing an adequate amount of omega-3s necessary for survival, these fatty acids are considered essential nutrients, mandating their acquisition through dietary sources or supplements.

One significant advantage of omega-3 fatty acids is their role in reducing triglyceride levels. These essential fats are integral to the composition of cell membranes throughout your body. Additionally, they serve as an energy source and play a vital role in maintaining the proper functioning of your heart, lungs, blood vessels, and immune system. DHA and EPA are specific types of omega-3s, primarily found in shellfish, while ALA is another variant found in plant sources. To incorporate more omega-3s into your diet, consider including foods such as fatty fish (e.g., salmon and mackerel), as well as incorporating flax seeds and chia seeds.

What are fatty acids?

Fatty acids serve as the fundamental components of the fats present in both our bodies and the foods we consume. During the process of digestion, fats are broken down into individual fatty acid molecules, which can then be absorbed into the bloodstream. Typically, fatty acid molecules are linked together in groups of three, forming a compound known as a triglyceride. The primary categories of fatty acids encompass saturated fats and unsaturated fats, with unsaturated fats further categorized into polyunsaturated fats and monounsaturated fats.

Fatty acids are chain-like chemical structures composed of

carbon, oxygen, and hydrogen atoms. The carbon atoms constitute the central structure of the chain, while oxygen and hydrogen atoms are attached at various points along it. Saturated fats lack any available attachment points, monounsaturated fats possess one such point, and polyunsaturated fats have multiple open attachment sites.

Saturated fats are often associated with health risks and are sometimes referred to as "unhealthy" or "bad" fats due to their potential to increase the likelihood of certain diseases such as heart disease and stroke. In contrast, unsaturated fats, including both polyunsaturated and monounsaturated fats, are considered "healthy" or "good" fats when consumed in moderation. Omega-3 fatty acids, a subset of polyunsaturated fats, represent a healthier choice in your diet compared to saturated fats.

Function of omega-3 fatty acids

Omega-3 fatty acids play a crucial role in promoting the proper functioning of all cells within the body. They are indispensable components of cell membranes, contributing to the structural integrity and facilitating intercellular interactions. While essential for all cells, omega-3s are notably abundant in cells of the brain and eyes.

Furthermore, omega-3s serve as a source of energy, supplying calories, and play a supportive role in maintaining the well-being of various bodily systems. These encompass the cardiovascular system and the endocrine system.

Types of Omega-3 fatty acids

There exist three primary categories of omega-3 fatty acids:

EPA (eicosapentaenoic acid) : EPA is among the various omega-3 fatty acids and is classified as a "marine omega-3" due to its presence in cold-water fatty fish like salmon. It is also a component of fish oil supplements, often in conjunction with docosahexaenoic acid (DHA).

DHA (docosahexaenoic acid) : DHA, another marine omega-3, is found in fish and is particularly vital for the growth and functional development of infants' brains.

ALA (alpha-linolenic acid) : ALA represents the plant-based form of omega-3 and is commonly found in sources like nuts, including walnuts. It plays an essential role in normal human growth and development.

Omega-3 fatty acids are indispensable nutrients that must be obtained through your diet. While the body can convert some of the ALA found in food into EPA and subsequently into DHA, this conversion process yields only a small quantity of EPA and DHA. Consequently, dietary sources of EPA and DHA, such as fish, are critical for meeting the body's omega-3 requirements.

Benefits of omega-3 fatty acids

Cardiovascular health

(n-3) Fatty acids have demonstrated specific cardiovascular benefits, which include reducing the risk of cardiac death caused by arrhythmias, lowering triglyceride levels, and exhibiting antithrombotic, anti-inflammatory, and antihypertensive effects. Research has shown that high-fat diets rich in (n-3) FAs, especially when compared to saturated fatty acids (SFAs), can mitigate dyslipidemia, decrease the release of cholesterol from arterial walls, suppress proinflammatory pathways in arterial walls, and increase anti-inflammatory markers in arterial walls. The concentration of circulating LDL and the types of fatty acids consumed in the diet can influence the arterial uptake of LDL. In addition to its role in hydrolyzing blood trigly-cerides, lipoprotein lipase (LpL) has a significant impact on LDL cell binding by acting as a bridge or anchor, facilitating the binding of LDL to the surface of macrophage cells, for example. Apart from the uptake of whole LDL particles, selective uptake, which involves the uptake of LDL cholesterol esters without the entire LDL particle, can lead to cholesterol deposition within cells and tissues like arterial walls, contributing to atherosclerosis.

In mouse models, a high-saturated fat diet significantly increases the supply of arterial cholesterol, mainly through a substantial increase in total LDL and selective uptake (more than fourfold). This increase is associated with elevated LpL and LpL activity in the arterial wall. Conversely, high-fat diets rich in (n-3) FAs markedly reduce selective uptake and greatly decrease the uptake of whole LDL particles, resulting in a decrease in LpL in the aortic media. However, there is a redistribution of LpL into the intima, which also demonstrates increased binding of LDL to the endothelial surface but no penetration of LDL into the arterial wall. As a result, it is plausible that (n-3) FAs reduce arterial cholesterol deposition by effectively anchoring LDL to the intimal surface, thereby inhibiting its penetration into deeper layers and, consequently, averting the development of atherosclerosis. In a recent comprehensive review, many mechanisms associated with the effects of (n-3) FAs on the arterial wall were extensively detailed.

Are omega-3 fatty acids good for you?

Consuming omega-3 fatty acids as part of your diet may reduce your risk of cardiovascular disease. Generally, it's preferable to obtain these essential nutrients from food sources, particularly fish, rather than relying on supplements.

While omega-3 dietary supplements, such as fish oil pills, can offer certain benefits to specific individuals, it's essential to exercise caution. Self-prescribing these supplements is not advisable. It's crucial to consult with your healthcare provider, whether it's your primary care physician or cardiologist, before considering over-the-counter (OTC) supplements. Your healthcare provider can prescribe dietary supplements based on your risk factors and lipid levels, as some supplements, depending on their dosage, can interfere with certain prescription medications.

- Elicit unpleasant side effects.
- Increase the risk of atrial fibrillation.
- Raise the risk of bleeding, especially if you're taking antiplatelet drugs or anticoagulants.

Moreover, different supplements contain varying formulations of omega-3 fatty acids, and not all of these formulations have demonstrated clear benefits for heart health. Promising research has primarily focused on a specific formulation known as icosapent ethyl, which is a purified form of EPA. This type of supplement may be beneficial for individuals meeting specific criteria, including those with diagnosed atherosclerotic cardiovascular disease, elevated triglycerides (135 to 499 milligrams per deciliter), and well-controlled LDL cholesterol levels (below 100 mg/dL) while taking statins.

Clinical trials examining the benefits of omega-3 supplements have yielded mixed results. Some studies suggest that these supplements can help protect the heart, while others show no significant advantage. These discrepancies may be attributed to variations in research methods, including dosage levels, omega-3 formulations, and the characteristics of the study participants.

As ongoing research continues to explore this topic, dietary guidelines and recommendations may evolve. Thus, it's crucial to engage in a dialogue with your healthcare provider, who can offer personalized advice based on your specific needs and medical history. The guidance they provide will be the most accurate, up-to-date, and scientifically supported information.

Best food sources of omega-3 fatty acids

Fish is the premier source of omega-3 fatty acids. The serving size for each fish type listed is 3 ounces (oz.), and the nutritional data is sourced from the U.S. Department of Agriculture. While a few fish varieties may contain a modest amount of ALA, the chart provides a consistent measure by presenting the combined DHA and EPA content. These figures represent the DHA and EPA content in uncooked (raw) fish, with exceptions clearly indicated where relevant.

What if I can't eat fish?

There are various reasons why fish may not be a part of your diet, such as allergies or adhering to a vegetarian or vegan lifestyle. In such cases, you can explore plant-based sources of omega-3, primarily in the form of ALA. Alternatively, you can consult with your healthcare provider to discuss the potential use of supplements like icosapent ethyl.

One of the most excellent sources of ALA is ground or milled flaxseed. Aim to incorporate around 2 tablespoons of it into your daily meals. You can easily achieve this by sprinkling it on items like oatmeal, smoothies, or yogurt.

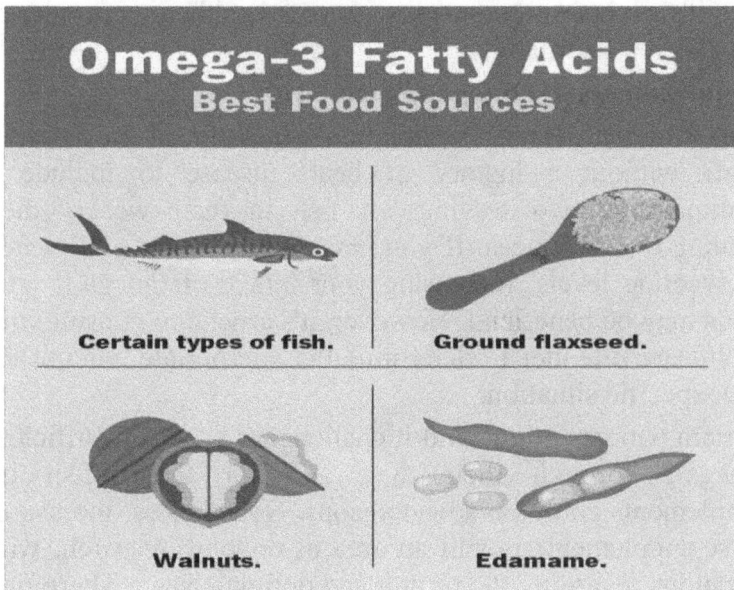

Omega-3 Fatty Acids
Best Food Sources

Certain types of fish.   Ground flaxseed.

Walnuts.   Edamame.

Other sources of ALA encompass:

Algae oil.

Canola oil.

Chia seeds.

Edamame.

Flaxseed oil.

Soybean oil.

Walnuts.

The recommended amount of ALA varies depending on several factors, including your age and assigned sex at birth.

Here are some general guidelines for adults :

Individuals assigned male at birth (AMAB): 1.6 grams.

Individuals assigned female at birth (AFAB): 1.1 grams.

Pregnant individuals: 1.4 grams.

Individuals who are breastfeeding (chest feeding): 1.3 grams.

To discover effective ways of incorporating ALA into your diet, it's advisable to consult with your healthcare provider or a registered dietitian.

Requirements of Omega -3 fatty acids

The American Heart Association generally advises individuals without a history of heart disease to include a minimum of two servings of fish in their weekly diet, totaling 6 to 8 ounces. If you have heart disease or elevated triglyceride levels, increasing your intake of omega-3 fatty acids may be beneficial. However, it's crucial to consult your healthcare provider to determine the appropriate amount for your specific situation.

Certain patients might find it challenging to obtain sufficient omega-3 through their diet, and for them, fish oil supplements could be advantageous. Nonetheless, the use of these supplements is still an area of ongoing research, with questions regarding the timing and optimal usage. Therefore, it's essential to use fish oil supplements only under the supervision and guidance of a healthcare professional.

References
1. Richard J. Deckelbaum, Claudia Torrejon. 2012.Health benefits of omega -3 fatty acids. The Journal of Nutrition, Volume 142, Issue 3, Pages 587S–591S, https://doi.org/10.3945/jn.111.148080
2. The Omega-3 Fatty Acid Nutritional Landscape: Health Benefits and Sources

Chapter- 4
Nutraceutical Properties in and around the Soybeans

Introduction

Functional foods are now widely available and rich in desirable bioactive components and high-quality nutrients thanks to current trends in healthy eating and lifestyles. Nutraceuticals with a high fibre, protein, and antioxidant potential can be found in some cultivated plants, like chia and soybeans, which are also excellent sources. The demand for animal feed, plant-based protein, and human nutritional needs are all driving the rapid growth of the soybean crop. Given the nutritious profile of soybeans, a variety of foods with soy as an ingredient are sold on the market.

In addition to being a lucrative oil crop, soybean (Glycine max Leguminosae) is a significant grain legume that is also utilised as aquaculture feed and as a feed for cattle. Although the origin and history of the soybean plant are unclear, ancient Chinese literature suggests that the Chinese emperor Sheng-Nung named soybeans after one of the five frightened grains as early as 2853 BC. The eastern section of northern China, which is said to be the soybean's original cultivation region, was where the crop was initially planted during the Shang era. For more than 4,000 years, China has grown soybeans. More than 35 countries cultivate soybeans for commercial purposes as a key oilseed. The United States produces 38% of the world's total soybean crop, followed by Brazil (25%), Argentina (19%), China (7%), India (3%), Canada (2%), and Paraguay (2%).The world's top producers of soy products are the United States, Brazil, Argentina, and India. Soybeans are native to China, and they are utilised extensively over the globe as a significant source of protein and edible oils.

Glycine and Soja are the two subgenera of the genus Glycine. The Glycine canescens and Glycine tomentella Hayata perennial wild species make up the first group. Asia's three annual species Glycine soja, Glycine gracilis, and Glycine max. Glycine soya is grown in China, Japan, Korea, Russia, and Taiwan, but Glycine max is grown exclusively in China. Glycine gracilis is also grown only in China. Soy is a prostrate, annual plant with pods, stalks, and leaves that are covered in tiny, brown or grey hairs. The trifoliate leaves have 3–4 leaflets per leaf and drop off before the seed reaches maturity. The expanding pod of the simple or curved soybean fruit is 3 to 7 cm long and contains one or two seeds. The mature seeds are light yellow, green, and brown in colour as opposed to the immature ones, which are green in colour. The most attractive colour for modern soybean cultivars is yellow and green, and they are spherical in shape. The papilionaceous type flowers are white, pink, and purple in colour. The soybean flower has a high level of self-pollination because the anthers ripen in the bud and discharge their pollen directly on the stigma of the same flower.

Soybean is a key ingredient in the production of oil, and the leftovers are fed to pets. Because soy includes a significant amount of protein (38–50%) and oil (18–25%), it has a high nutritional value and is a widely consumed food. In Western nations, both soy product production and consumption have increased. Soybeans are used in both fermented and unfermented foods in Asian countries, including soy sauce, miso, natto, yoghurt, kinako, protein crisps, sweets, and soy milk, which is then converted into tofu, aburage, and yuba. They are also used to make infant food. For a variety of conditions, including lactose intolerance and acute gastroenteritis in babies, soy products are utilised as the main source of protein. About 35% protein, 31% carbs, 17% fat, 5% minerals, and 12% moisture are found in ripe soybeans.

Histidine, isoleucine, leucine, lysine, phenylalanine, tyrosine, threonine, tryptophan, and valine are among the necessary amino acids found in soy protein that are acceptable amounts and should be consumed daily as part of a balanced diet. It has been claimed that soy provides a number of health advantages, including reducing plasma cholesterol, improving bone mineral density, and protecting against intestinal and kidney illnesses. Isoflavones, saponins, proteins, and peptides found in soybeans are responsible for these health advantages.

Soy products

Foods made from soybeans can be divided into unfermented and fermented foods. Unfermented foods include – tofu, soymilk, edamame, soy nuts and sprouts, while fermented soy products include – miso, tempeh, natto and soy sauce.

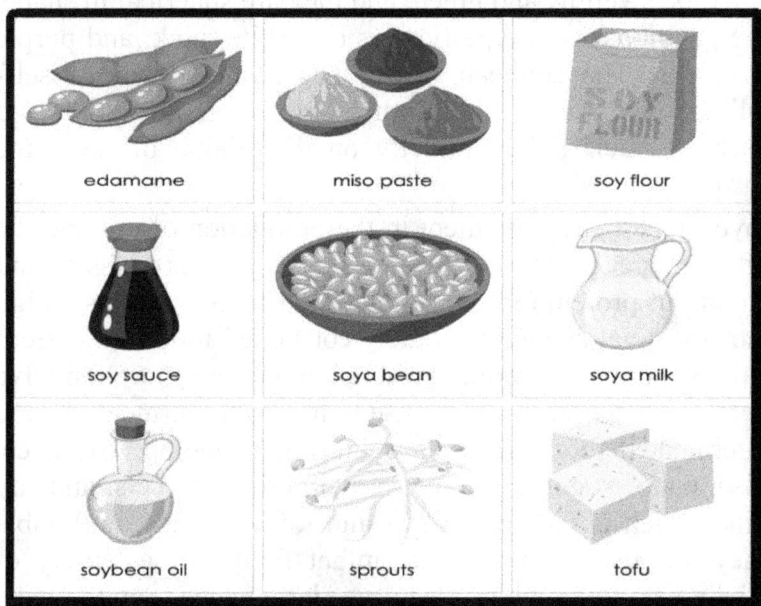

Figure:1 pictorial representation of different products of soya bean

Nutritional component

Protein: soya contains 35-40% protein by dry weight, including globulins, 11S glycinin and 7S β-conglycinin .These proteins contain all the amino acids essential for human nutrition, making soy products nearly equivalent to animal sources in protein quality, but with less saturated fat and no cholesterol. Soy also contains the biologically active protein components hemagglutinin, trypsin inhibitors, α-amylase and lipoxygenase. According to the FDA's "Protein Digestibility Corrected Amino Acids" procurement method, soybeans are not only high-quality protein, but are now believed to play preventive and therapeutic roles for various diseases .The Comparative analysis of amino acid composition (mg/g) of egg, milk and soy protein are mentioned below (Table 1):

Amino acid	Egg protein[a]	Milk protein[a]	Soy protein[b]
Cysteine	24	7.9	13.1–35.1
Threonine	47.8	47.3	14.9–45.2
Valine	48.2	63.8	16.8–42.1
Isoleucine	51.4	68.5	14.6–40.2
Leucine	82.9	103.5	43.5–73.3
Lysine	66.4	68.3	46.8–137.8
Methionine	34.9	20.2	12.4–53.7
Phenylalanine	59.5	46.7	24.9–50.2
Histidine	23.5	21.8	27.3–58.7

[a] Source: FAO. Accessed at: www.fao.org/docrep
[b] Values for soy protein are from the 44 soybean lines that are presented as a range

Table 1: Comparative analysis of amino acid composition (mg/g) of egg, milk and soy protein

Oil: About 19% of soybeans are oil, with triglycerides making up the majority of the oil. In terms of total fatty acids, soybean oil has comparatively high levels of polyunsaturated fatty acids (PUFA), including 51% linoleic acid, 8% -linolenic acid, 4% stearic acid, 10% palmitic acid, and 23% oleic acid. Linoleic acid and -linolenic acid, which are essential fatty acids that belong to the -6 and -3 families and are found in soybean oil, are crucial for controlling a number of metabolic pathways as well as performing critical nutritional and physiological functions. Additional components of the oil include 1-3% phospholipids, 35% phosphatidylcholine, 25% phosphatidylethanolamine, 15% phosphatidyl inositol, and 5- 10% phosphatidic acid.

Carbohydrates: Stachyose (4%) and raffinose (1.1%) are two examples of the oligosaccharides present in soybeans, which make up around 35% of their total carbs. When compared to raffinose, which is a triose with a galactose-glucose-fructose structure, stachyose is a tetrase. Fibre from insoluble sources makes up the majority of polysaccharides. Polysaccharides that dissolve in galacturonic acid can be found in soybean curd waste (Okara). Soluble polysaccharides have been utilised to alter the physical attributes of many meals in addition to their usage as a dietary fibre supplement.

Vitamins and Minerals: Soy is a better source of B vitamins than cereals, while being deficient in vitamin B12 and C. Soybean oil contains tocopherols as well, potent natural antioxidants. Soy has a 5% mineral content as well. The contents of K, P, Ca, Mg, and Fe are all quite high. Soy ferritin is a suitable source of iron supplements.

Effect of soy in various disease conditions
❖ **Coronary heart disease**
According to certain investigations, soy-based products with healthful proteins have a substantial effect. Numerous studies have provided an explanation for the variations in death rates from various forms of cancer and cardiovascular disease (ECV) in various nations based on a holistic dietary

and nutritional approach. A number of studies have shown that casein and other animal proteins are more atherogenic and better at decreasing cholesterol than their plant-derived counterparts. People with normal or high cholesterol levels may significantly lower their cholesterol levels by consuming soy protein. Use of soy isoflavones has been shown to improve cardiovascular conditions and lower cardiovascular disease risk factors in women and men after early menopause. As a preventative measure for cardiovascular symptoms, blood pressure imbalance can happen as a critical event in many cardiovascular diseases. The antihypertensive action of peptides generated from Lactobacillus fermented soybean milk, The results showed that with the increase in peptide levels, there is a reduction in systolic blood pressure and may be the explanation for maintaining low blood pressure control.

❖ **Bone health:**
Soybeans are a simple approach to build strong bones and even lower your risk of osteoporosis. They are a fantastic source of protein and calcium. According to research, the isoflavones, genistein, and daidzein found in soybeans help to reduce bone loss and fractures. Additionally, soy protein keeps our bodies' calcium levels stable. Folic acid, which is found in soy, works in concert with other nutrients to stop bone loss. A class of naturally occurring chemical compounds known as isoflavones belongs to the isoflavonoids family. The additional subclasses of flavonoids, in addition to isoflavones, include flavonols, aurones, flavones, flavanols, chalcones, and the red and blue anthocyanin colours. Isoflavones are 1,4-benzopyrone rings with the phenyl ring B connected at position 3. The highest concentration of isoflavones (up to 3 mg g-1 dry weight) can be found in soy.

❖ **Anticancer effects**
A cancerous growth of cells that remains in one place or

spreads further across the body. Different diets Materials rich in nutrients have anticancer properties and are effective in preventing a number of malignancies. Human colon cancer cell lines HT-29 and Caco-2 were effectively suppressed in vitro by fermented soy milk beverages. Using fermented soy milk, studies have been conducted on the reduction of the production and development of reactive oxygen species in mice with MCF-7 oestrogen receptor-positive human breast cancer.The regulation of MMP (matrix metallopeptidase) levels and the prevention of cancer can both be significantly influenced by the diet of soybeans and products derived from them.

Only a few reports of peptides with antitumor potential have been made, despite numerous studies on fermented soybeans with anticancer and anticancer characteristics. The peptides synthesised during the breakdown of soy protein, surfactants (which contain cyclic peptide), or lipopeptides produced by the starting culture can all contribute to the anticancer activities of fermented soybean peptides. In numerous experimental systems, soy peptides have also been found to possess anticancer effects. The murine lymphoma cell cycle G2/M phase progression was stopped by the purified hydrophobic peptide X-MLPSYSPY from defatted soy protein (P388D1). Numerous investigations have shown that the majority of soy peptides with anticancer characteristics come from the minor group 2S fraction of soy protein.

Due to their potential to prevent cancer, soy isoflavones have received a lot of attention over the years. Soy isoflavones have been described as dietary substances that may play a part in reducing the emergence of several cancer kinds, such as breast and prostate cancer tumours. Animal studies have indicated that the main isoflavone in soybeans, genistein, is beneficial at preventing the development of cancer. Numerous studies show that genistein inhibits the growth of human cancer cells by altering the expression of genes involved in the control of the cell cycle and apoptosis. Activation of the NF-B and Akt signalling pathways, which are known to maintain a homeostatic balance between cell survival and apoptosis, has also been found to be effectively inhibited by genistein. Genistein has been shown to block NF-B translocation dimer to the nucleus and its binding to DNA, preventing transcription of NF-B downstream genes.In general, oestrogen receptor interaction has been linked to the antiproliferative effects of soy isoflavones.Different concentrations of isoflavones and various breast tumour cells have been used in studies to examine how these compounds affect apoptosis, cell growth and survival, antioxidant capabilities, or the suppression of angiogenesis and metastasis.

❖ **Reduce neonatal mortality**

Folate is essential for one-carbon metabolism, which controls gene expression, cell division, the synthesis of neurotransmitters, and amino acid metabolism, as well as the physiological synthesis of nucleic acids. Folic acid can lower neonatal mortality caused by neural tube defects. Through folic acid fortification and supplementation, folic acid has a protective effect against the risk of newborn mortality. health and disease implications of folic acid supplementation throughout pregnancy. The nutrient folate may lower the risk of heart disease. Due to the influence of folate, there is considerable debate over the existence of various health effects during pregnancy.

On a dry matter basis, soy contains about 2500 g kg-1 of folic acid. There is room to investigate the folic acid content and bioaccessibility in processed wheat and its derivatives. Folic acid levels are negatively impacted by processing conditions. Numerous other health issues, including anaemia, nutrient malabsorption, child brain development, Alzheimer's disease treatment, age-related hearing loss, etc., have been linked to folic acid. Soybeans are a strong source of this vitamin, thus diets high in them may be useful for nutrition.

❖ **Antidiabetic effects**

Diabetes mellitus (DM), a metabolic disorder, is one of the most significant health issues in the world today. There are currently 336 million people in the world, and by 2030, that number is expected to rise to 552 million.For the treatment of DM, a number of meals made of phytocompounds are available. These include soybeans, which have demonstrated noteworthy results in the prevention of DM.Patients with chronic renal disease have benefited significantly by dietary soy, which has been proven to be vital. Diabetes mellitus is frequently associated with severe renal disease. When used as an animal protein alternative in type 1 diabetes, soy protein lowers both proteinuria and GFR.

Isoflavonoids have been added to soy products, which shows how they have an anti-diabetic impact. Soybean extract has also been shown to be effective in preventing the brush border membrane's vesicles from absorbing glucose.As a potential target of glucose transporter 4 (GLUT4), stigmasterol from soybean oil has been examined for its anti-diabetic properties. In vitro and in vivo research has been done on stigmasterol (SMR), which has been shown to have antidiabetic effects. The phytosterol stigmasterol, which is generated from edible soybean oil, has been shown to have a considerable impact on the management of type 2 diabetes mellitus. Chungkookjang, a fermented soybean product from Korea made up of smaller peptides and isoflavonoid glycones, has also been investigated for its improved insulinotropic action in the islets of type 2 diabetic rats. In alloxan-induced diabetic rats, oral testing for the anti-diabetic effects of fermented soybean and flaxseed milk (FSFM) was conducted. improved probiotic milk that has been fermentedthe effectiveness of isoflavones in the management of type 2 diabetes. Flaxseed with soy milk

46

shown its effectiveness in lowering type 1 diabetes without causing any side effects.

Antioxidant effects

An imbalance between free radicals and antioxidant mechanisms leads to oxidative stress. continue as The primary mechanism in a multitude of illnesses like diabetes, cancer, etc. In terms of reducing oxidative stress and scavenging free radicals, soy and its derivatives are particularly effective. On soy and its products' antioxidant capacity, numerous investigations have been done. Dou-chi, a conventional cuisine made of soy and fermented with an Aspergillus species, shown the capacity to dislodge scavenger radicals. In the study, different phenols and flavonoids were isolated, and one of them was 3'-hydroxydaidzein, which has strong 2,2-diphenyl-1-picrylhydrazyl (DPPH) free radical scavenging properties. Inhibiting oxidative stress in type 2 diabetes mellitus (T2DM) in humans, soy milk is a crucial soy product. According to research, fermented soy milk is helpful in regulating levels of total antioxidants, oxidised glutathione, 8-isoprostaglandin F2, glutathione peroxidase, malondial-dehyde, and reduced glutathione (GSH), as well as in enhancing oxidative activity stress in T2DM. By using gel filtration and Sephadex G-15 chromatography, antioxidant peptides were extracted from fermented soybean protein flour hydrolyzate and showed significant antioxidant activity. Creation of highly nutrient-dense fermented soy meals components and biologically relevant characteristics were also examined. The nutritional components of fermented soybeans, including their fatty acids, isoflavones, and amino acids, as well as their antioxidant ability against ABTS [2,2'-azino-bis (3-ethylbenzothiazoline-6-sulfonic acid), DPPH, and hydroxyl radicals, were observed to have changed by Lee et al. They also examined the fluctuations in total phenol content, the impacts of -glucosidase, and the inhibitory action of glucosidase.

S.No.	Soy component	Applications	Molecular mechanism
1.	Isoflavones	Anti-cancerous, anti-fibrosis, anti-estrogen, osteoporosis, anti- artherosclerosis, type 2 diabetes, anti-oxidant, neuro-protection etc.	Form complexes with ER receptors because of structural similarities with estrogens, thus modulating estrogen receptor signalling pathways.
2.	Bioactive peptides	Antioxidative, anti-hyper-sensitive, anti-cancerous, anti-diabetic, immunostimu-latory, anti-obesity.	Act as competitive inhibitors for enzymes responsible for diabetes and synthesis of cholesterol (di peptidyl peptidase-IV, HMG Co-A reductase etc).
3.	Saponins	Anti-inflammaotory, antimi-crobial, anti-carcinogenic, cardio protective effects.	Form complexes with cholesterol and inhibit their absorption in intestine and also cause inhibition of tumour associated enzymes and hormone receptors.
4.	Protease inhibitors	Antiproliferative	Inhibit activities of trypsin, chymotrypsin, chymase, mitogen activated protein kinase. Also downregulate the protease activities, playing major role in cancer.

Table 2: Applications and molecular mechanism of various soy components

Source : Garima et al., 2020

References:

1. Garima Dukariya, Shreya Shah, Gaurav Singh and Anil Kumar (2020) Soybean and Its Products: Nutritional and Health Benefits. J Nut Sci Heal Diet 1(2): 22-29.
2. P. Singh, K. Krishnaswamy,Sustainable zero-waste processing system for soybeans and soy by-product valorization,Trends in Food Science & Technology,Volume 128,2022,Pages 331-344,ISSN 0924-2244, https://doi.org/10.1016/j.tifs.2022.08.015
3. Shashank A. Tidke, D. Ramakrishna, S. Kiran, G. Kosturkova and G.A. Ravishankar, 2015. Nutraceutical Potential of Soybean: Review. *Asian Journal of Clinical Nutrition, 7: 22-32.*

4. Valentina V. Nikolić*, Slađana M. Žilić, Marijana Z. Simić, Vesna A. Perić. Maize Research Institute, Zemun Polje, 11185 Belgrade – Zemun, Slobodana Bajića 1, SerbiaBLACK SOYA Bean And Black Chia Seeds As A Source Of Nutrients And Bioactive Compounds With Health Benefits, Food and Feed Research Journal of the Institute of Food Technology, University of Novi Sad UDK 633.34+633.883]:664.641.2:613.26, ISSN: 2217-5369 (print), 2217-5660 (online edition) 2020, 47, 2

Chapter- 5

Ginger for different Disease Condition

Introduction

The well-known herbaceous plant ginger (Zingiber officinale Roscoe) has been used for a long time as a flavouring and herbal remedy. Additionally, taking ginger rhizome as a supplement is a normal traditional treatment for ailments like pain, nausea, and vomiting. In particular, a significant number of randomised clinical studies (RCTs) have been carried out to investigate the antiemetic impact of ginger in a number of circumstances, including motion sickness, pregnancy, and post-anesthesia.

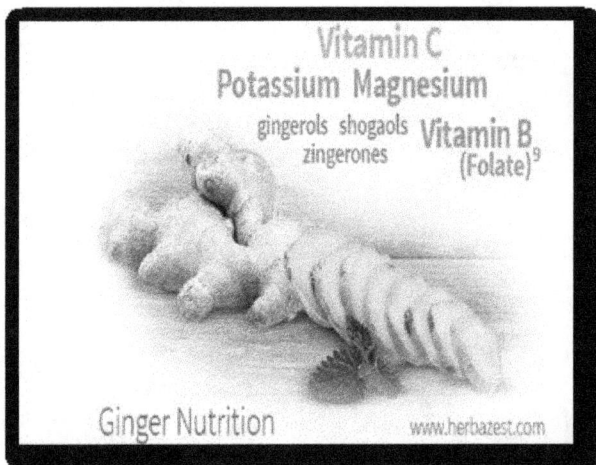

From ginger, more than 100 different chemicals have been identified. The principal chemical classes in ginger are specifically gingerol, shogaol, zingiberene, and zingerone. Other less prevalent chemical classes include terpenes, vitamins, and minerals. The nutritive value of ginger is mentioned below (Table 1&2). Ginger (Zingiber officinale) is a spice that offers a range of nutritive components, including vitamins, minerals, and bioactive compounds.

While ginger is often used in relatively small quantities for flavoring, it can still contribute to your overall nutrient intake. Here's an overview of the nutritive value of ginger:

1. Vitamins :

• **Vitamin B6 :** Ginger contains a small amount of vitamin B6, which is important for brain health, metabolism, and immune function.

• **Vitamin C:** Ginger provides a modest amount of vitamin C, an antioxidant that supports the immune system and skin health.

2. Minerals :

• **Potassium :** Ginger contains potassium, an essential mineral that helps regulate fluid balance, muscle contractions, and nerve signals.

• **Manganese :** Ginger is a good source of manganese, a trace mineral involved in bone health, metabolism, and antioxidant defense.

3. Dietary Fiber :

Ginger contains dietary fiber, which is beneficial for digestive health and can contribute to a feeling of fullness.

4. Bioactive Compounds :

• **Gingerols :** These bioactive compounds are responsible for ginger's distinctive flavor and aroma. Gingerols have antioxidant and anti-inflammatory properties and are believed to contribute to many of ginger's potential health benefits.

• **Shogaols :** Formed from gingerols when ginger is dried or cooked, shogaols also possess antioxidant and anti-inflammatory effects.

• **Zingerone :** This compound is responsible for the spicy taste of ginger and has potential antioxidant and anti-inflammatory properties.

• **Gingerdiols** : Emerging research suggests these compounds may have anti-diabetic potential.

Table 1: Proximate composition ginger root raw

Nutritional value of Ginger root raw

Serving Size: 0.25 Cup, 24 g

Calories 19 Kcal.	Calories from Fat 1.62 Kcal.	
Proximity	**Amount**	**% DV**
Water	18.93 g	N/D
Energy	19 Kcal	N/D
Energy	80 kJ	N/D
Protein	0.44 g	0.88%
Total Fat (lipid)	0.18 g	0.51%
Ash	0.18 g	N/D
Carbohydrate	4.26 g	3.28%
Total dietary Fiber	0.5 g	1.32%
Total Sugars	0.41 g	N/D

Table 2: Mineral composition ginger root raw

Minerals	Amount	% DV
Calcium, Ca	4 mg	0.40%
Iron, Fe	0.14 mg	1.75%
Magnesium, Mg	10 mg	2.38%
Phosphorus, P	8 mg	1.14%
Potassium, K	100 mg	2.13%
Sodium, Na	3 mg	0.20%
Zinc, Zn	0.08 mg	0.73%
Copper, Cu	0.054 mg	6.00%
Manganese, Mn	0.055 mg	2.39%
Selenium, Se	0.2 µg	0.36%

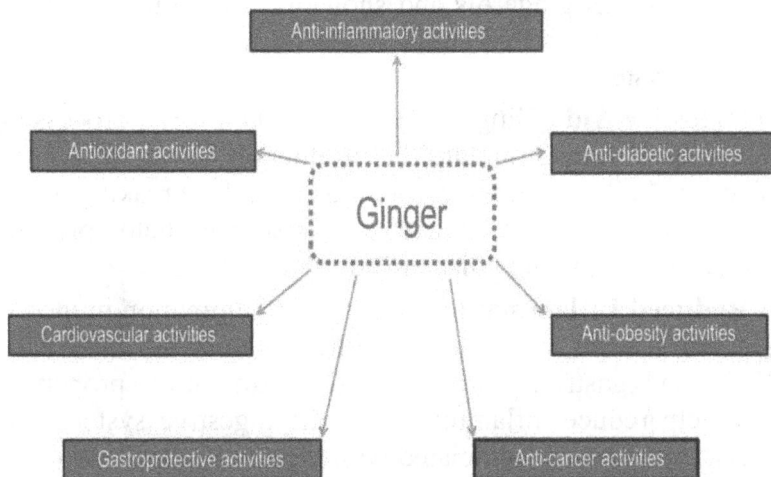

Figure 1: Pictorial presentation of nutrition implication of ginger

Clinical Effects of Ginger

❖ Antiemetic Function

Patients who had the first cycle of mildly to severely emetogenic chemotherapy and had CINV (chemotherapy-induced nausea and vomiting) found that ginger considerably improved quality of life. In addition, ginger successfully decreased both acute and late CINV in both children and adults.In severe circumstances, nausea and vomiting of pregnancy (NVP), also known as hyperemesis gravidarum, is a frequent pregnancy symptom that can result in nutritional deficiency. Ginger is more effective than vitamin B6 at reducing the severity of nausea. In spite of this, ginger might help gynaecological patients.

❖ Gastrointestinal function

a) Relief from Nausea and Vomiting : Ginger is perhaps most well-known for its ability to alleviate nausea and vomiting. It has been used as a natural remedy for motion sickness, morning sickness during pregnancy, and chemotherapy-induced nausea. The active compounds in ginger, such as gingerols and shogaols, are thought to have anti-nausea effects by acting on the GI tract and the central nervous system.

b) Digestive Aid : Ginger can promote the overall process of digestion. It may stimulate the production of saliva, gastric juices, and bile, all of which are important for breaking down food and absorbing nutrients. This can help prevent indigestion and related discomfort.

c) Reduced Inflammation : Chronic inflammation in the GI tract can lead to conditions like inflammatory bowel disease (IBD) and gastritis. Ginger's anti-inflammatory properties may help reduce inflammation in the digestive system and alleviate symptoms associated with these conditions.

d) Relief from Gastrointestinal Discomfort : Ginger is known for its soothing properties that can help ease various forms of GI discomfort, including bloating, gas, and abdominal pain. It may help relax the intestinal muscles, providing relief from spasms and cramps.

e) Improved Gut Motility : Ginger may support healthy gut motility, which is the movement of food and waste through the digestive tract. This can contribute to regular bowel movements and prevent constipation.

f) Protection of Gastric Lining : Some research suggests that ginger may have a protective effect on the stomach lining, potentially reducing the risk of gastric ulcers by inhibiting the growth of Helicobacter pylori bacteria and promoting mucus production.

❖ **Inflammatory effect**

Ginger (Zingiber officinale) has been studied for its potential anti-inflammatory effects, and several components of ginger are believed to contribute to these properties. Here's how ginger may play a role in reducing inflammation:

a) **Anti-Inflammatory Compounds** : Ginger contains bioactive compounds called gingerols, which have been shown to possess anti-inflammatory properties. These compounds may inhibit various pathways involved in inflammation by modulating the expression of inflammatory genes and enzymes.

b) **Cytokine Modulation** : Ginger may help regulate the production and release of pro-inflammatory cytokines, which are signaling molecules that play a central role in the inflammatory response. By modulating cytokine production, ginger may help reduce excessive inflammation.

c) **COX and LOX Inhibition** : Gingerols in ginger have been reported to inhibit enzymes such as cyclooxygenase (COX) and lipoxygenase (LOX), which are involved in the synthesis of pro-inflammatory prostaglandins and leukotrienes, respectively. By inhibiting these enzymes, ginger may help lower inflammation.

d) **Oxidative Stress Reduction** : Ginger possesses antioxidant properties, which means it can help neutralize harmful molecules called free radicals that contribute to oxidative stress and inflammation. By reducing oxidative stress, ginger may indirectly lower inflammation.

e) **Immune System Regulation** : Ginger may help modulate the immune response by influencing immune cell activity and the release of immune-related molecules. This can contribute to a balanced immune reaction and potentially reduce chronic inflammation.

❖ **Metabolic enhancement**

Substantial drops in fasting blood sugar, insulin sensitivity, and insulin resistance are all effects of ginger on diabetes-related indices like glycemic indicators, lipid levels, and blood pressure. The lowering of C-reactive protein, triglycerides (TG), low-density lipoprotein cholesterol (LDL), -C), and malondialdehyde showed that ginger consumption also had an impact on the lipid profile, inflammatory markers, and antioxidants. Ginger supplementation reduced insulin and the HOMA-IR (homeostasis model assessment of insulin resistance) and increased the QUICKI (quantitative sensitivity assessment index to all insulin). Ginger has been shown to be helpful in lowering cardiovascular risk factors associated with obesity, including body fat mass, body fat percentage, total cholesterol, waist circumference, waist-hip ratio, and insulin resistance. Additionally, ginger may have antioxidant and antimetabolic effects on obese breast cancer patients. The overall consensus was that ginger may help lower the risk factors for metabolic disorders.

❖ **Effects of antioxidant stress**

Free radicals created by biological systems are scavenged by components of ginger's rich phytochemistry. A certain type of free radical produced during oxidation is necessary for the synthesis of energy. Oxidative stress, which can result in DNA damage, is brought on by an increase in free radical production.For the organism to remain healthy under such unbalanced conditions, supplementation with extra antioxidants through dietary modules is crucial. In several in vitro and in vivo studies, the antioxidant capabilities of ginger and its constituents have been investigated. Humans will surely be protected against a wide range of chronic diseases if antioxidant level is improved within the body. The inclusion of certain alpha, beta unsaturated ketones is what gives ginger its strongest anti-inflammatory and antioxidant capabilities. According to animal studies, ginger considerably lowers induced lipid peroxidation and raises blood glutathione levels in addition to antioxidant enzyme levels. Additionally, malathion-induced lipid peroxidation in rats receiving malathion (20 ppm) for 4 weeks was greatly reduced by feeding the animals 1% weight/weight ginger. The GSH-dependent enzymes glutathione peroxidase, gluta-thione reductase, and glutathione S-transferase were all considerably reduced when ginger (1% w/w) was fed concurrently with lindane. Zingerone decreased lipid peroxidation in vitro, eliminated O2- and OH, and may be helpful in treating Parkinson's disease.

Superoxide dismutase, catalase, glutathione peroxidase, glutathione reductase, and glutathione levels in liver tissue were all considerably decreased by ethanol. Treatment of rats with 1% dietary ginger for a month increased this impact, indicating that ginger may act as a preventative measure against ethanol-induced hepatotoxicity. In renal failure, ginger and gum arabic have demonstrated renoprotective benefits. These protective effects can be linked to its anti-inflammatory qualities by decreasing serum C-reactive protein levels as well as antioxidant effects by lowering lipid peroxidation marker, malondialdehyde levels, and enhancing renal superoxide dismutase activity. In order to stop the progression of the disease and postpone the requirement for renal replacement treatment, they may be an advantageous supplementary therapy for patients with acute and chronic renal failure.

❖ **Anticancer effects**

Several components found in ginger, including [6]-gingerol, [6]-shogaol, [6]-paradol, and zerumbone, have anti-inflammatory and anticancer properties. Colorectal, gastric, ovarian, hepatic, cutaneous, mammary, and prostatic cancer can be effectively controlled with ginger and its bioactive components.

Vegetarians are more likely to develop colorectal cancer, and ginger may help stop the disease's development. Colon cancer development can be inhibited by ginger supplementation, which can activate several enzymes including glutathione peroxidase, glutathione-S-transferase, and glutathione reductase.

Apoptosis-inducing ligand linked to tumour necrosis factor (TRIALS) is crucial in encouraging apoptosis in gastric cancer. Ginger and its useful constituents trigger cascades of caspase protein. Hepatoma cell invasion and proliferation can both be inhibited by gingerol. The major causes of gingerol in these tumour cells are cell cycle arrest and activation of apoptosis. In rats with liver cancer, ginger extract can lower the increased production of TNF-alpha and NF-B. Ginger works to treat skin cancer by preventing angiogenesis in mouse skin. Through the apoptosis-mediated suppression of human squamous cell growth brought on by reactive oxygen species (ROS), gingerol demonstrated exceptional cytotoxicity.

Inhibiting NF-B activation and lowering VEGF and IL-8 release are two ways ginger works to cure ovarian cancer. Ginger can treat breast cancer by preventing cell adhesion and invasive motility. By altering proteins connected to the apoptotic pathway, gingerol can have an impact on models of prostate cancer.

❖ **Antidiabetic effects**

Ginger (Zingiber officinale) has been investigated for its potential anti-diabetic effects, and while research is ongoing, some studies suggest that ginger may offer benefits for managing diabetes. Here are some ways in which ginger may play a role in anti-diabetic activity:

a) Blood Sugar Regulation : Ginger may help improve insulin sensitivity and enhance glucose uptake by cells. Insulin sensitivity is a key factor in diabetes management, as it allows cells to efficiently utilize glucose from the bloodstream. By enhancing insulin sensitivity, ginger may contribute to better blood sugar control.

b) Pancreatic Function : Some studies suggest that ginger may have a protective effect on pancreatic beta cells, which are responsible for producing insulin. Preserving the function of these cells can help maintain insulin production, which is essential for regulating blood sugar levels.

c) Anti-Inflammatory Effects : Chronic inflammation is associated with insulin resistance and type 2 diabetes. Ginger's anti-inflammatory properties may help reduce inflammation in tissues and organs involved in glucose metabolism, contributing to improved insulin sensitivity.

d) Antioxidant Activity : Ginger contains antioxidants that can help counteract oxidative stress, which plays a role in the development and progression of diabetes. By reducing oxidative stress, ginger may help protect against diabetic complications.

e) Glycemic Control : Some research suggests that ginger may slow the absorption of glucose from the digestive tract, leading to a more gradual rise in blood sugar levels after meals. This can contribute to better glycemic control, particularly after eating carbohydrate-rich meals.

f) Lipid Profile Improvement : Diabetes is often associated with dyslipidemia (abnormal lipid levels). Ginger consumption has been linked to improvements in lipid profiles, including reductions in total cholesterol, triglycerides, and LDL cholesterol, which are important factors in diabetes management.

g) Weight Management : Maintaining a healthy weight is crucial for diabetes management. Ginger has been studied for its potential role in supporting weight loss and reducing obesity-related inflammation, which can indirectly benefit individuals with diabetes.

References:
1. Anh, N. H., Kim, S. J., Long, N. P., Min, J. E., Yoon, Y. C., Lee, E. G., Kim, M., Kim, T. J., Yang, Y. Y., Son, E. Y., Yoon, S. J., Diem, N. C., Kim, H. M., & Kwon, S. W. (2020). Ginger on Human Health: A Comprehensive Systematic Review of 109 Randomized Controlled

Trials. *Nutrients*, *12*(1),157.
https://doi.org/10.3390/nu12010157.
2. Bioactive Compounds and Bioactivities of Ginger (Zingiber officinale Roscoe). Priyadarshini, K., & Gupta, A. (2019). Bioactive Compounds and Bioactivities of Ginger (Zingiber officinale Roscoe). *Pharmacognosy Reviews*, 13(26), 1-19. doi:10.4103/pr.pr_227_18
3. Ginger on Human Health: A Comprehensive Systematic Review of 109 Randomized Controlled Trials. Zhang, Y., Zhang, L., & Li, Q. (2020). Ginger on Human Health: A Comprehensive Systematic Review of 109 Randomized Controlled Trials. *Evidence-Based Complementary and Alternative Medicine*, 2020, 9977249. doi:10.1155/2020/9977249
4. Gingerols and shogaols: Important nutraceutical principles from ginger. Kapoor, V., & Kapoor, S. (2015). Gingerols and shogaols: Important nutraceutical principles from ginger. *Current Pharmaceutical Design*, 21(41), 6241-6253. doi:10.2174/1381612821666150908110317
5. Mashhadi, N. S., Ghiasvand, R., Askari, G., Hariri, M., Darvishi, L., & Mofid, M. R. (2013). Anti-oxidative and anti-inflammatory effects of ginger in health and physical activity: review of current evidence. *International journal of preventive medicine*, 4(Suppl 1), S36–S42
6. Nutraceutical Potential of Ginger. Kumar, A., & Kumar, S. (2021). Nutraceutical Potential of Ginger. *Advances in Food & Nutrition Research*, 109, 1-16. doi:10.1016/bs.afnr.2021.01.001

Chapter -6

Carotenoids as Nutraceutical

Introduction

Carotenoids are biosynthesized by bacteria, algae, fungi, and plants (the majority of which can be found in higher plants, particularly their leaves, flowers, and fruits), but not by animals, which must obtain them from diet. These are a set of around 700 naturally occurring pigments that are biosynthesized by plants, algae, fungus, and bacteria. These compounds are classified into two groups based on their structural elements: carotenes, which are composed of carbon and hydrogen (for example, -carotene, -carotene, and lycopene), and xanthophylls, which are composed of carbon, hydrogen, and oxygen (for example, lutein, -cryptoxanthin, zeaxanthin, astaxanthin, and fucoxanthin). Carotenoids have several beneficial effects on human health, including pro-vitamin A effect, antioxidant, anticancer, anti-obesity, and anabolic action on bone components.

Carotenoids are currently employed as feed additives, animal feed supplements, natural food colours, nutritional supplements, and, more recently, nutraceuticals for cosmetic and pharmacological applications. Chemical techniques can be used to commercially generate these substances. Synthesis, fermentation, or isolation from a limited number of readily available natural sources. Furthermore, commercial production of carotenoids from microbes competes mostly with synthetic production via chemical synthesis. However, the majority of commercial carotenoids (for example, -carotene, astaxanthin, and canthaxanthin) are created through chemical synthesis.

Carotenoids are compounds composed of C5 eight isoprene linked in a head and tail pattern, with the majority of them containing 40 carbon atoms. These chemicals are formed from phytoene, which is produced through the dimerization of geranylgeranyl pyrophosphate (GGPP) via a reductive mechanism. Flow chart 1: Schematic diagram of the carotenoid biosynthesis pathway in plants.

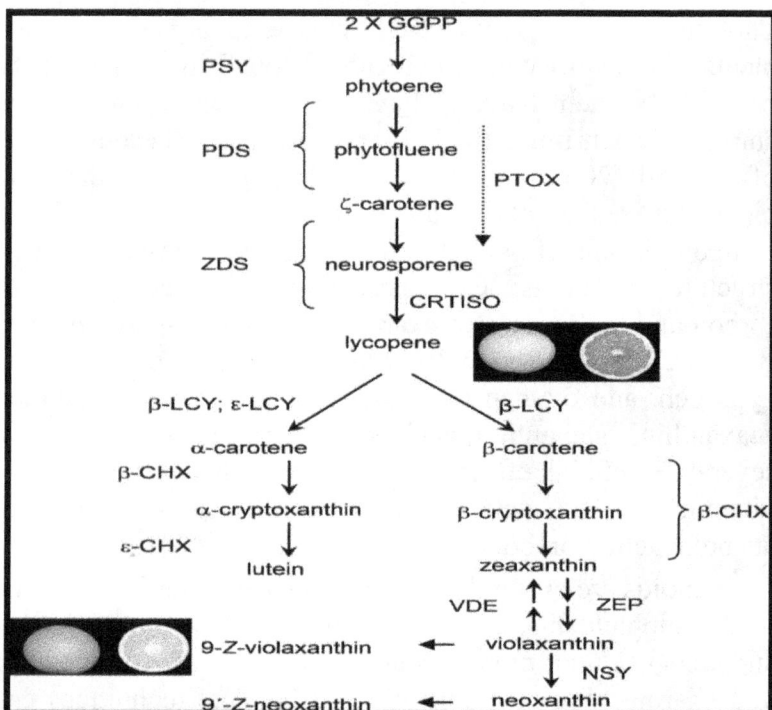

Carotenoids are structurally divided into two main classes:

❖ Carotenes (for example, a-carotene, b-carotene, lycopene), which are exclusively hydrocarbons (those without any oxygen molecule)

❖ xanthophylls (for example, lutein, zeaxanthin, fucoxanthin and astaxanthin) which are oxygenated containing hydroxyl, methoxy, carboxyl, keto or epoxy resin.

Carotenoids perform vital biological roles in nature as auxiliary components for light harvesting of photosynthetic systems, photoprotective antioxidants, and membrane fluidity regulators, as well as being responsible for the distinctive colours of diverse fruits and vegetables. These molecules, which are responsible for the spectrum of colours ranging from bright yellow to orange to dark red, are biosynthesized in all photosynthetic organisms, including cyanobacteria, algae, and higher plants, as well as some bacteria, yeasts, and non-photosynthetic fungi. Carotenoids, as light collection pigments, serve an important function in protecting plants from excessive light and photooxidative stress. Carotenoids also include a lengthy core chain of conjugated double bonds with acyclic or cyclic substituents.

❖ Carotenoids are intracellular products that are typically found in the membranes of mitochondria, chloroplasts, or the endoplasmic reticulum. Carotenoids are generally very hydrophobic substances, therefore they are found in lipids (oil, fat) or in hydrophobic structures such as membranes. Carotenoids from fruits, vegetables, and animals are typically fat soluble and connected with lipid fractions, lipid parts of human tissues, cells, and the lipid core of the membrane bilayer. The orientation of a single carotenoid in the membrane and its effect on membrane properties are determined by structural factors such as carotenoid size and shape, as well as the presence of functional groups.

Sources of Carotenoids
Carotenoids are produced by bacteria, algae, fungus, and plants, but not by animals, who must receive them through their diet. Carotenoids generated by microorganisms include lycopene, -carotene, astaxanthin, lutein, zeaxanthin, -cryptoxanthin, and canthaxanthin, as well as vegetables (Table 1), fruit, grains, and so on. The most prevalent in human plasma are lycopene, -carotene, lutein, zeaxanthin, and -cryptoxanthin.

➢ β -cryptoxanthin is a carotenoid pigment present in citrus fruits such as orange and mandarin. This carotenoid is prevalent in Satsuma mandarin (Citrus unshiu MARC) and is converted enzymatically in plants from -carotene.

➢ Lycopene is the pigment that gives tomatoes, red grapes, watermelon, and rose grapefruit its red colour. It can be seen on papayas and apricots as well. Lycopene is present in our food, most notably in tomatoes and tomato products.

➢ Zeaxanthin is the dihydroxy form of beta-carotene and is found in a variety of foods, including maize and vegetables. Zeaxanthin is a yellow-colored oxygenate carotenoid or xanthophyll that occurs naturally in cornflowers, alfalfa, and calendula. This also contains a lot of zeaxanthin. Wolfberry contains a high concentration of zeaxanthin, which is found in goji berries. This chemical has been employed in the cosmetics, bird feed, pigs, and fish industries. Beta-carotene was extracted and identified from Canarium odontophyllum Miq seeds peel, pulp, and fractions. In addition, microalgae, Dunaliella salina, and Flavobacterium produced -carotene and zeaxanthin.

➢ Astaxanthin is a red pigment present in Red Sea creatures such as crabs, prawns and goldfish (such as Red Sea sea bream and salmon). At the moment, astaxanthin is primarily produced through chemical synthesis, but some processes for biological astaxanthin production have been developed using natural sources such as green algae Haematococcus pluvialis and yeast Xanthophyllomyces dendrorhous (formerly classified as Phaffia rhodozyma). Fucoxanthin is found in common foods such as seaweed and is one of the main carotenoids found in marine species. Carotenoids can also be found in colourful fruits and vegetables such as apricots, melon, carrots, pumpkin, and sweet potato, which include-carotene and -carotene.

Table 1: Common Dietary Sources of Carotenoids in Fruits and Vegetables

Food	β-Carotene	Lutein	β-Cryptoxanthin	Lycopene	α-Carotene	Zeaxanthin
Carrot	7975	271	-	-	2186	-
Spinach	4489	6265	-	-	-	-
Broccoli	1580	2560	-	-	-	-
Lettuce	890	1250	-	-	-	-
Green peas	548	1840	-	-	-	-
Watercress	5919	10713	-	-	-	-
Tomato	608	77	-	4375	-	-
Orange*	250	120	700	-	200	-
Orange juice*	375	1180	1980	-	-	-
Mandarin*	275	50	1775	-	-	140
Sweet corn	45	520	-	-	60	440
Red pepper*	1700	270	250	-	30	600
Apricot*	3500	70	120	trace	Trace	-
Mango*	3100	-	800	-	-	-
Papaya*	640	-	770	3400	30	-
Watermelon	180	20	300	4750	trace	-

Note: *: carotenoid esters present. Source: Southon and Faulks (2003).

Lycopene, beta-carotene, phytofluene, and phytoene are found in pink grapefruit, tomatoes, and watermelon. Spinach has lutein, zeaxanthin and beta-carotene; mango, papaya, peaches, plums, squash, and oranges include lutein, zeaxanthin, cryptoxanthin, and beta -carotene, phytofluene, and phytoene. However, no specific values are provided; instead, the content is indicated as a range, as seen below; Low: 0 to 0.1 mg/100 g; medium: 0.1 to 0.5 mg/100 g; high: 0.5 to 2 mg/100 g; extremely high: >2 mg/100 g.

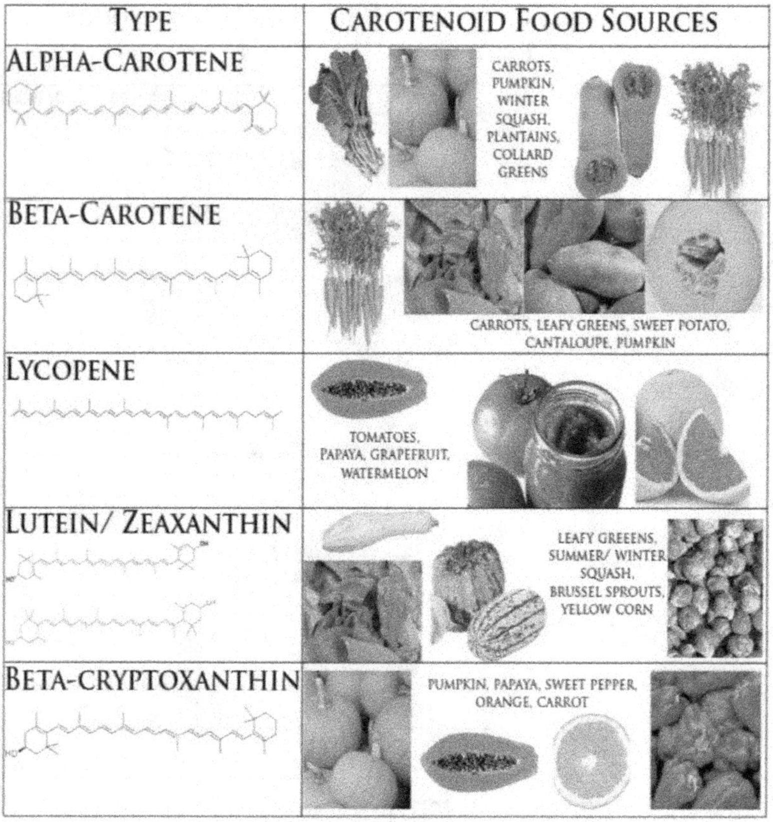

TYPE	CAROTENOID FOOD SOURCES
ALPHA-CAROTENE	CARROTS, PUMPKIN, WINTER SQUASH, PLANTAINS, COLLARD GREENS
BETA-CAROTENE	CARROTS, LEAFY GREENS, SWEET POTATO, CANTALOUPE, PUMPKIN
LYCOPENE	TOMATOES, PAPAYA, GRAPEFRUIT, WATERMELON
LUTEIN/ ZEAXANTHIN	LEAFY GREEENS, SUMMER/ WINTER SQUASH, BRUSSEL SPROUTS, YELLOW CORN
BETA-CRYPTOXANTHIN	PUMPKIN, PAPAYA, SWEET PEPPER, ORANGE, CARROT

SOURCE: USDA DATABASE FOR FLAVONOID CONTENT OF SELECTED FOODS

Figure 1: Schematic representation of different sources of carotenoids

Health Benefits of Carotenoids are as follows
➤ **Eye Health**
Carotenoids such as provitamin A Indeed, the provitamin A activity of carotenoids was known for a long time. More than 600 natural carotenoids have been identified. Of the approximately 700 naturally occurring carotenoids, only about 50 have them provitamin A activity , among these, only three are the most important Vitamin A precursors in humans: α-carotene, β-carotene and β-cryptoxanthin   which

are converted into vitamin A or retinol in the body. β-carotene is the main one provitamin A component of most carotenoids foods and is found in fruits and vegetables, is a weel nutrient known to exhibit pro-vitamin A activity . This compound is a precursor of vitamin A, which is well known to be able to prevent serious eye injuries diseases, such as night blindness. Also, to function physiologically like vitamin A, carotenoid-containing foods should be fine digested to release carotenoids from the food matrix.

❖ **Carotenoids as antioxidants/pro-oxidants**

Carotenoids can operate as antioxidants in all species and promote resistance to oxidative stress in the human body; carotenoids are part of the antioxidant defence. Carotenoids, like tocopherols, can extinguish simple oxygen. Carotenoids and tocopherols are recognised to be potent antioxidants capable of eliminating reactive oxygen species formed under photo-oxidation stress. Carotenoids can also eliminate oxidising free radicals via at least three processes (Equations 1–3) involving their addition, electron transfer, and addition and transfer of hydrogen atoms. They can also directly react with superoxide and other free radicals. Carotenoids (CAR) can arise by methods centred on resonance stabilised carbon radicals, such as interaction with lipid peroxyl radicals.

One of the best-documented mechanisms is that singlet oxygen ($1O_2$, lycopene) does not get enough energy to cause excitation of other molecules, resulting in the generation of reactive species. That is why a single lycopene molecule can quench several free radicals. Lycopene, unlike other carotenoids, has no pro-vitamin A characteristics; however, due to its unsaturated form, it is regarded a powerful antioxidant and singlet oxygen quencher. Carotenoids, particularly lycopene and -carotene, are excellent single oxygen ($1O_2$) fire extinguishers in photosensitized oxidation. The lycopene concentration of tomatoes varies greatly depending on the type and ripeness of the tomato. Lycopene, the most abundant carotenoid in tomatoes, has the highest antioxidant activity of any dietary carotenoids. Cooking and food processing increase lycopene bioavailability by increasing the lipophilic compound's accessibility for the synthesis of lipid micelles with dietary lipids and bile acids. As a result, lycopene absorption is greater after consuming processed tomatoes (tomato pasta) than after consuming fresh tomatoes. Also, in addition to lycopene, β-carotene and other carotenoids have antioxidant properties in vitro and in animal models. The use of animal models for the study of carotenoids is limited since most animals they do not absorb or metabolize carotenoids in a similar way to humans. Subsequently, reported that the antioxidant activity of lycopene. It has been shown that α-carotene is superior to that of β-carotene. Also, carotenoid blends or combinations with other antioxidants (for example, vitamin E) can increase its activity against free radicals.

❖ **Carotenoids as anticancer agents**

Worldwide, there are approximately 10 million cancer diagnoses each year. Year and the number is rapidly increasing. Was predicted that if people ate plant-based diets rich in on a variety of vegetables (broccoli, carrots, rocket, pumpkins, sweet potatoes, courgettes, tomatoes, watercress) and fruits (apricots, melons, mangoes, papayas, peaches and persimmons, legumes) minimally processed starchy staple foods every day, the overall cancer rates could drop by up to 20% . A diet that includes enough amount of fruits and vegetables, including what they are rich in carotenoids, it is scientifically compatible low risk strategy that would allow the possible beneficial effects of carotenoids on cancer risk and progression done.

Carotenoids (α-carotene, lutein, zeaxanthin, lycopene, β-cryptoxanthin, fucoxanthin, astaxanthin), as well as β-carotene, may be beneficial for cancer prevention. Scientific interest in dietary carotenoids has has increased in recent years due to its benefits effects on human health, such as reducing the risk of cancer and improved immune system function, which are attributed to its antioxidant potential.

A diet that includes enough vegetables (broccoli, carrots, arugula, squash, sweet potatoes, squash, tomatoes, watercress) and fruit (apricots, melons, mangoes, papayas, peaches and persimmons, legumes), including those rich in carotenoids, is a scientifically sustainable low-risk compound strategy that would allow the possible beneficial effects of carotenoids on cancer risk and progression done. In this sense, the scientific interest on dietary carotenoids (α-carotene, lutein, zeaxanthin, lycopene, β-cryptoxanthin, fucoxanthin, astaxanthin), such as just like β-carotene has increased in recent years because of its beneficial effects on human health, such as reduce the risk of cancer and improve the immune system function of the system, which are attributed to its antioxidant power Among carotenoids, lycopene is the main component found in serum. Interestingly, it has been shown that the carotenoid (lycopene) has been shown to enhance connexin expression43, a gene encoding major gap junction protein and hence Up-regulated Gap Crossing communication. and acted like anticancer. lutein, Zeaxanthin and cryptoxanthin are the main xanthophylls carotenoids in human plasma. The consumption of these xanthophylls is directly associated with the reduction of risk of cancer, cardiovascular disease, age-related macular degeneration and cataract formation.

❖ **Carotenoids as an anti-obesity effect**

Obesity is an abnormal condition produced by lipids accumulation in adipose tissue. Around the internal organs is an important risk factor that causes many kinds of diseases. Many Interest has focused on the adaptive thermogenesis of uncoupling protein (UCP) families (UCP1, UCP2, and UCP3) as a physiological defense against obesity, hyperlipidemia and diabetes. Mitochondrial uncoupling protein 1 (UCP1), usually expressed only in brown adipose tissue (BAT), is a key molecule for anti-obesity as his dysfunction contributes to the development of obesity. Feeding with fucoxanthin (carotenoid) significantly reduce white adipose tissue (WAT) in rats and mice with clear expression of UCP1 protein and mRNA in WAT, while there was little expression of UCP1 in WAT mice fed a control diet. Also, the combination of fucoxanthin and fish oil were more effective in attenuating WAT weight gain versus fucoxanthin feeding alone. Hence, the daily intake of fucoxanthin in mice also caused a significant reduction body weight.

Furthermore, astaxanthin inhibits body weight gain and the weight of adipose tissue caused by a high-fat diet. In addition, astaxanthin reduced the weight of the liver, the liver triglycerides, plasma triglycerides and total cholesterol. These results indicated that astaxanthin could be beneficial in the prevention of obesity. Carotenoid as anabolic effect on bone components β-Cryptoxanthin is a type of carotenoid which has a potential effect on maintaining bone health and on prevention of osteoporosis. The presence of β-cryptoxanthin (10-7 or 10-6 M) caused a significant increase in calcium alkaline phosphatase content and activity in femoroshaft and femorometaphyseal tissues in 50-week-old female rats. This compound can have a stimulating effect on bone loss that induces osteoporosis leading to bone fracture, its oral administration induced an anabolic effect on bone components in femoral tissue of aged female rats in vivo.

Furthermore, this carotenoid has a powerful anabolic effect on bone calcification in the femorodiaphyseal (cortical bone) and rat femoro-metaphyseal (trabecular bone) in vitro and in vivo. Furthermore, the intake of fortified juice, which contains more β-cryptoxanthin than regular juice, has a preventive effect on bone loss with age. Moreover, reported that prolonged intake of fortified juice with β-cryptoxanthin it has a stimulating effect on the bone formation and an inhibitory effect on bone resorption in humans, which is useful in menopausal women.

References

1. Aoki H, Kien NTM, Kuze N, Tomisaka K, Chuyen NV (2002). Carotenoid Pigments in GAC Fruit (Momordica cochinchinensis SPRENG). Biosci. Biotechnol. Biochem., 66(11): 2479-2482.
2. Bonnie TYP, ChooYM (1999). Oxidation and Thermal degradation of carotenoids. J. Oil Palm Res., 2(1): 62-78.
3. Carrillo-Lopez A, Yahia EM, Ramirez-Padilla GK (2010). Bioconversion of Carotenoids in Five Fruits and Vegetables to Vitamin A Measured by Retinol Accumulation in Rat Livers. Am. J. Agric. Biol. Sci., 5(2): 215-221.
4. Chang RCC, Ho YS, Yu MS, So KF (2010). Medicinal and nutraceutical uses of wolfberry in preventing neurodegeneration in Alzheimer.
5. Mattea F, Martin A, Cocero MJ (2009). Carotenoid processing with supercritical fluids. J. Food Eng., 93: 255-265.
6. Sugawara T, Yamashita K, Asai A, Nagao A, Shiraishi T, Imai I, Hirata T (2009). Esterification of xanthophylls by human intestinal Caco-2 cells. Arch. Biochem. Biophy., 483: 205-212.
7. Yamaguchi M (2008). β-cryptoxanthin and Bone Metabolism: The Preventive Role in Osteoporosis. J. Health Sci., 54(4): 356-369.
8. Southon S, Faulks R (2003). Carotenoids in food: bioavailability and functional benefits. In: Phytochemical functional foods. Johnson, I and Williamson, G (Eds.). Ch. 7. Woodhead Publishing Limited. CRC Press. ISBN 0-8493-1754-1, pp. 107-127

9. Irwandi, J., Dedi, N., Reno, F. H., and Fitri, O.,(2011), Review Carotenoids: Sources, medicinal properties and their application in food and nutraceutical industry, Journal of Medicinal Plants Research Vol. 5(33), pp. 7119-7131, http://www.academicjournals.org/JMPR

Multiple uses of Dietary Fibres as Nutraceuticals in different Disease Conditions

Introduction

Dietary fibre is a group of food components which is resistant to digestive enzymes and found mainly in cereals, fruits and vegetables. Dietary fiber and whole grains contain a unique blend of bioactive components including resistant starches, vitamins, minerals, phytochemicals and anti-oxidants. Dietary fiber which indigestible in human small intestinal, on the other hand digested completely or partially fermented in the large intestine, is examined in two groups: water-soluble and water insoluble organic compounds. Dietary fiber can be separated into many different fractions. These fractions include arabinoxylan, inulin, pectin, bran, cellulose, β-glucan and resistant starch. Dietary fibres compose the major component of products with low energy value that have had an increasing importance in recent years. Dietary fibres also have technological and functional properties that can be used in the formulation of foods, as well as numerous beneficial effects on human health. Dietary fibre components organise functions of large intestine and have important physiological effects on glucose, lipid metabolism and mineral bioavailability.

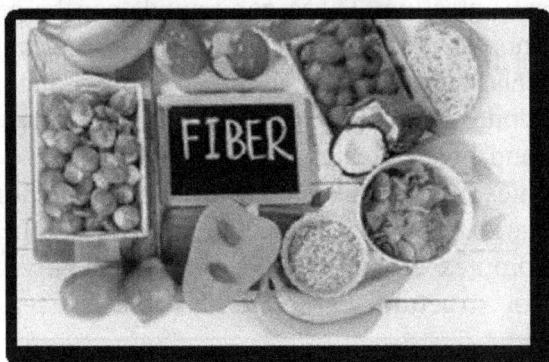

Defining Dietary Fiber

A recent description was suggested by the American Association of Cereal Chemists, terms dietary fiber as carbohydrate polymers with more than a three degree polymerization which are neither digested nor absorbed in the small intestine. The greater than three degree polymer rule was designed to exclude mono and disaccharides.

The World Health Organization (WHO) and Food and Agriculture Organization (FAO) agree with the American Association of Cereal Chemists (AACC) definition but with a slight variation. They state that dietary fiber is a polysaccharide with ten or more monomeric units which is not hydrolyzed by endogenous hormones in the small intestine. The known constituents of dietary fiber are listed in Table 1. Non Starch Polysaccharides (NSP) can be further subdivided into the two general groups of soluble and insoluble. Most fiber containing foods include approximately one-third soluble and two-third insoluble fiber.

Grouping of Carbohydrates

In the simplest form, carbohydrates can be separated into two basic groups based upon their digestibility in the Gastro Intestinal (GI) tract.

❖ The first group (i.e. starch, simple sugars, and fructans) is easily hydrolysed by enzymatic reactions and absorbed in the small intestine. These compounds can be referred to as non-structural carbohydrates, non-fibrous polysaccharides (NFC) or simple carbohydrates.

❖ The second group (i.e. cellulose, hemicellulose, lignin, pectin and beta-glucans) are resistant to digestion in the small intestine and require bacterial fermentation located in the large intestine. These compounds can be referred to as complex carbohydrates, non-starch polysaccharide (NSP) or structural carbohydrates and are reflective in

Neutral Detergent Fiber (NDF) and Acid Detergent Fiber (ADF) analysis.

- NSP can be further subdivided into the two general groups of soluble and insoluble. This grouping is based on chemical, physical, and functional properties.

- Soluble fiber dissolves in water forming viscous gels. They bypass the digestion of the small intestine and are easily fermented by the microflora of the large intestine. They consist of pectins, gums, inulin-type fructans and some hemicelluloses.

- In the human GI tract, insoluble fibers are not water soluble. They do not form gels due to their water insolubility and fermentation is severally limited. Some examples of insoluble fiber are of lignin, cellulose and some hemicelluloses.

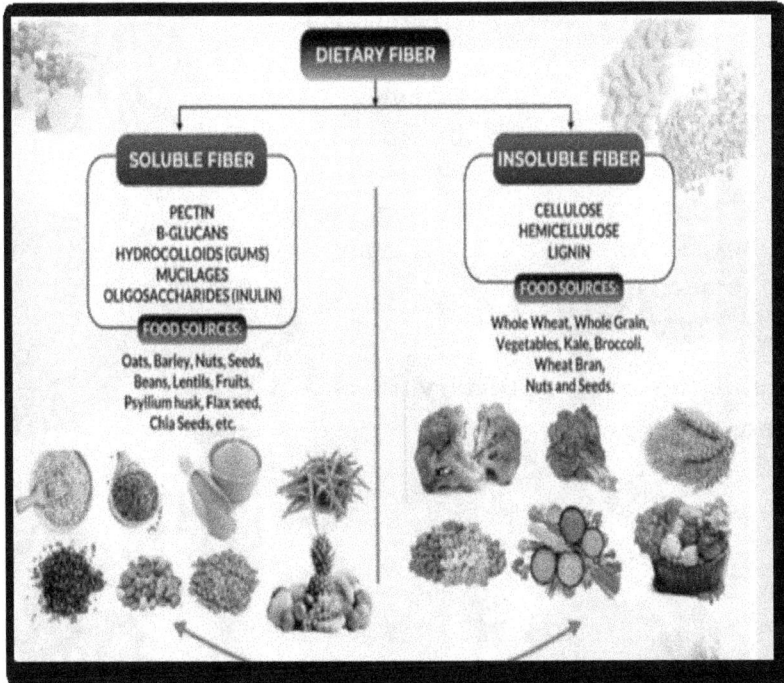

Table 1. Components of dietary fiber according to the American Association of Cereal Chemists

Non-Starch polysaccharides and oligosaccharides	Analogous carbohydrates	Lignin substances associated with the NSP and lignin complex
Cellulose	indigestible dextrins	Waxes
Hemicellulose	resistant maltodextrins	Phytate
Arabinoxylans	resistant potato dextrins	Cutin
Arabinogalactans	synthesized carbohydrates compounds	saponins
Polyfructoses	Polydextrose	Suberin
Inulin	methyl cellulose	Tannin
Oligofructans	hydroxypropylmethyl cellulose	
Galacto-oligosaccharides	resistant starches Gums	
mucilages, pectins		

Table 2. Sources of Dietary fibers

Materials	Soluble dietary fiber	Insoluble dietary fiber	Total dietary fiber
Nori	16.8	17.9	34.7
Whole soy	7.08	65.24	72.32
Whole wheat	2.87	41.59	44.46
Whole corn	0.40	87.47	87.87
Rice	0.19	0.75	0.94

Beans	10.85	25.64	36.49
Chickpeas	1.35	16.69	18.04
Onion	3.59	13.32	16.89
Potatoes	2.14	4.85	6.99
Apricot	26.43	44.92	71.35
Peaches	27.30	39.53	66.83
Apples	18.56	55.57	74.13
Spinach, cooked	0.6	3.5	4.1
Field beans, cooked	2.1	9.3	11.4
Broad beans,cooked	0.8	7.3	8.3
Bitter gourd	3.1	13.5	16.6
Green plantain,100g	0.2	5.8	6.0
Flaxseed	10.15	12.18	22.33
Beetroot	2.4	5.4	7.8
Cluster beans	0.6	6.1	6.7
Carrot	1.6	4.1	5.7
Fenugreek leaves	0.7	4.2	4.9
Ladyfingers	1.3	3.0	4.3
Almonds	1.10	10.10	11.20
Sesame seeds	1.90	5.89	7.79
Brazil nuts	1.30	4.10	5.40

Health Benefits of Dietary Fiber as nutraceuticals.

Obesity

Epidemiological studies provide information that dietary fiber, especially consumption of grains or cereal fiber helps to protect against the increase of obesity. Various mechanisms have been suggested for how dietary fibers have a positive effect on management of weight; reduce assimilation of macronutrients, and also changing secretion of hormones from the gut. A large number of observational studies showed the contrary, and frequently dose-dependent, the correlation between fiber consumption and body weight.

Howarth et al. found that higher consumption of dietary fiber has been related to weight loss of about 2 kg over 4months. Increase consumption of dietary fiber may decrease absorption of energy by the method of diluting a diet's availability of energy while maintaining other essential nutrients. The ability of management of body weight of dietary fibers could be attained by various factors like it may considerably decrease intake of energy and diet metabolizable energy; fermentation of soluble fiber in the large intestine produces glucagon-like peptide (GLP-1) and peptide YY (PYY), which is act as inducing satiety. Soluble and insoluble fiber may help in losing body weight. However, there is a relationship between the fat content of diet and type of fiber used in consumption

Dietary fiber's ability to decrease body weight or attenuate weight gain could be contributed to several factors. First, soluble fiber, when fermented in the large intestine, produces glucagon-like peptide (GLP-1) and peptide YY (PYY). These two gut hormones play a role inducing satiety. Second, dietary fiber may significantly decrease energy intake [Tucker and Thomas 2009]. Women who consumed increased levels of fiber tended to also have a decreased consumption of dietary fat. Third, dietary fiber may decrease a diet metabolizable energy (ME), which is gross energy minus the energy lost in the feces, urine and combustible gases. Baer et al. [1997] observed that an increased consumption of dietary fiber resulted in a decrease in the ME of the diet. This may be attributed to the fact that fat digestibility decreased as dietary fi ber increased. Also, as dietary fiber intake increases, the intake of simple carbohydrates tends to decrease. Although, dietary fiber still contributes to the total caloric content of a diet, it is much more resistant to digestion by the small intestine and even somewhat resistant in the large intestine.

Both soluble and insoluble fiber may lead to weight loss. However, there seems to be a relationship between the type of diet (high or low fat) and the type of fiber consumed. Insoluble fiber may play a more important role for weight loss during consumption of a high fat diet. Since resistant starch is a constituent of dietary fiber and undergoes the same digestion as insoluble fiber, comparing resistant starch and insoluble fiber may give us a better understanding of how dietary fiber can be used to treat and prevent obesity. Adding resistant starch to a diet dilutes its ME, but not to the degree of insoluble fiber. Numerous studies have found the same inverse relationship between dietary fiber and weight gain .

Immunity

Inulin and other oligofructoses have been the most extensively studied dietary fibers. They act, to stimulate growth of bifidobacteria in the colon. Bifidobacteria and lactobacilli are health promoting bacteria that generate short-chain fatty acids and stimulate the immune system. Fairly extensive animal studies have documented the favourable effect of inulin on the immune system and preliminary studies in humans support the hypotheses generated from animal studies. Inulin and oligofructoses are not digested by pancreatic enzymes thus, they enter the colon virtually intact. In the colon, inulin is fermented completely by the microbacteria and it promotes the growth of bifidobacteria. Short-chain fatty acids (SCFA) result from this fermentation process. Other fibers are also fermented to generate SCFA, but the bifidobacteria effects of non-oligofructose fibers are not as well characterised. The proposed health benefits of bifidobacteria include the following:

- protection from intestinal infection
- lowering of intestinal pH for formation of acids after assimilation of carbohydrates
- reduction of the number of potentially harmful bacteria; production of vitamins and antioxidants
- activation of intestinal function and assistance in digestion and absorption, especially of calcium • bulking activity to prevent and treat constipation
- stimulation of the immune response
- potential reduction in the risk for colorectal cancer.

Limited studies in humans have indicated that inulin supplementation increases the fecal bacterial contents of bifi dobacteria and has favourable effects on the types and amounts of circulating lymphocytes. Inulin and oligofructoses have been studied most extensively, but favourable effects of fermentable soluble fi bers have been demonstrated for oat b-glucan, gumArabic, and others. The role of prebiotic fi bers in infant nutrition and health, especially for non-breastfed infants, is generating a great deal of interest. The studies suggest that supplementation with a prebiotic fi ber mixture has the following benefi ts: promotes postnatal immune development, decreases respiratory infections and atopic dermatitis and improves bowel function. The therapeutic potential for using prebiotic fi bers in the treatment of infl ammatory bowel disease is being examined. In animal studies, prebiotic fi bers have reduced gut infl ammation in a number of animal experimental models. Early studies also indicate that prebiotic fi bers signifi cantly reduce the risk of infection in liver transplant patients. Preliminary human studies have shown favourable responses for individuals with ulcerative colitis, Crohn's disease, or pouchitis .

Cardiovascular

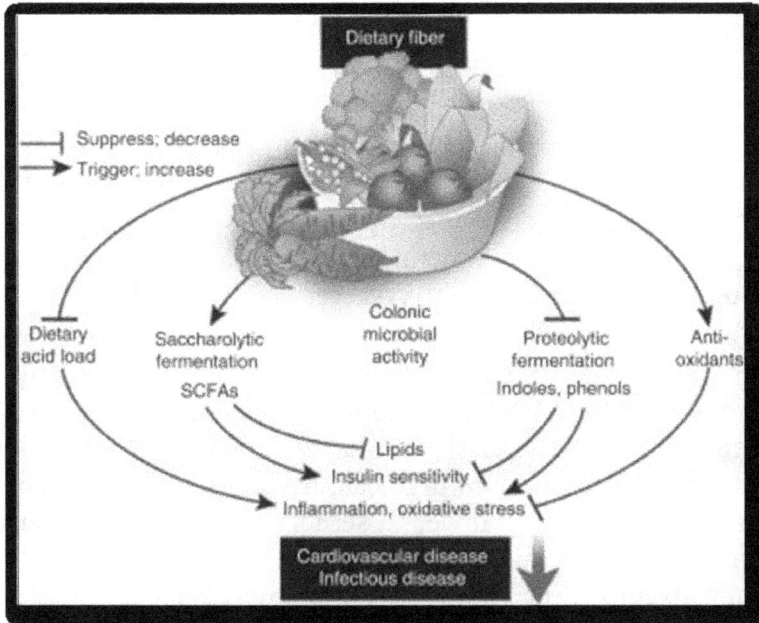

Cardiovascular diseases, including coronary heart disease (CHD), stroke, and hypertension, affect more than 80 million people and are the leading causes of morbidity and mortality in the United States. In 2005, CHD was the leading cause of death and strokes were the third leading cause of death in the United States. While CHD is the most prevalent cause of death, it is probably the most modifi able; an estimated 82% of CHD is attributed to lifestyle practices such as diet, physical activity, and cigarette abuse and 60% is attributed to dietary patterns . High levels of dietary fi ber intake are associated with meaningfully lower prevalence rates for coroner heart disease, stroke, and peripheral vascular disease.

In a long term clinical study, Jensen et al. [2004] reported that an increased daily consumption of bran signifi cantly decreased the risk of coronary heart disease in healthy adult men. This is most likely due to the data reported by Qureshi et al. [2002] who found that 10 g of rice bran consumed for eight weeks was able to decrease serum total cholesterol, LDL cholesterol and triglycerides. The mechanisms behind these effects may be twofold. The reduction in cholesterol levels is likely due to an increase in bile acid synthesis. Andersson et al. [2002] found that oat bran doubled the serum concentration of 7α-hydroxy-4-cholesten-3-one (α-HC), which is a metabolite in the synthesis of bile acids that is oxidized from 7α-hydroxycholesterol. The reduction in serum triglyceride levels may be a result of a decreased absorption of fat from the small intestine.

Theuwissen and Mensink [2008] found that, many well-controlled intervention studies have shown that four major water-soluble fiber types β-glucan, psyllium, pectin and guar gum effectively lower serum LDL cholesterol concentrations, without affecting HDL cholesterol or triacylglycerol concentrations. Furthermore, epidemiological studies suggest that a diet high in water-soluble fiber protects against CVD. These findings underlie current dietary recommendations to further increase water-soluble fiber intake

Diabetes

Two type of diabetes has been seen in patients from last decades i.e. Type I and Type II. It was found that total carbohydrates had no significant effect on the risk of diabetes in patients. Carbohydrates having higher glycemic index could be considered as it produces higher blood glucose concentrations while those with a low glycemic index result in a lesser glucose/insulin response. Weickert and Pfeifer stated that an enlarged intake of fiber from cereals significantly improved whole-body glucose disposal. A study has concurred that dietary fibers obtained from whole cereal grains have a significant decrease in the occurrence of diabetes but fruits or vegetables dietary fiber had no significant effect on the risk of diabetes. Higher intake of insoluble dietary fiber from cereal was powerfully linked with remarkably reduce diabetes risk. It can also be concluded that insoluble fiber may reduce appetite and food intake, it could lead to decreased in caloric and body mass index. Several studies have verified affirmative physiological effects of both soluble and insoluble dietary fiber offer physiological benefit mainly by lowering the blood cholesterol and reduce intestinal absorption of glucose. A Meta-analysis has been done by intervention trials using high fiber product (18.3 g/d) in type 2 diabetic patients and it reveals that FPG and HbA1c were moderately reduced by 0.83mmol/l and 0.26%, respectively, when compared with control. However, these results show that these soluble and insoluble fibers play a vital role in the prevention of diabetes.

Gastrointestinal and Colonic Fermentation

Gastrointestinal tract (mouth to anus) is also affected by consumption of dietary fibers. Fiber-rich foods generally take a longer time to eat and have low energy density. Fermentation occurs to all the dietary fibers to the same extent but soluble dietary fibers are more fermentable. In the colon, these fibers increase bacterial mass and some of them act as prebiotics which developed health-promoting bacteria like Lactobacillus and bifidobacteria. Fermentability of dietary fiber also plays a very vital role in the reduction of diabetes risk. Soluble fibers typically impediment gastric emptying and also slowed down the transit of food throughout the small intestine. Recent studies showed that oral supplementation of pectin to the infants and children having diarrhea showed the positive effect and reduces acute intestinal infections. Researchers also suggested that consumption of dietary fiber reduces the occurrence of peptic ulcer disease, hiatal hernias and gastroesophageal reflux disease (GERD), appendicitis, gallbladder disease, colorectal cancer, hemorrhoids and diverticular disease.

Higher consumption of dietary fiber is generally used for the avoidance and management of constipation and irritable bowel syndrome. Wheat bran and fiber-rich cereals are used by consumers, which showed beneficial effects.

Cancer

Cancer continues to be one of the number one health concerns of populations worldwide. Most cancers strike both men and women at about the same rate, with exception of cancers of the reproductive system. Of particular concern is cancer of the colon, ranking among the top 3 forms of cancer in the U.S.A., for both men and women. Colon cancer is also one of the leading causes of cancer morbidity and mortality among both men and women in the Western countries, including the U.S.A. Historical observational and epidemiological studies from around the world have long supported that increased consumption of fruits and vegetables and high fiber intake provide a protective relationship between dietary fiber intake and colon cancer incidence. Early results from a European investigation, the European Prospective Investigation of Cancer (EPIC), involving more than half a million people in 10 European countries, indicates that dietary fiber provides strong protective effects against colon and rectal cancers. Poorly fermented fiber, such as that in cereal brans, has direct effects in the colon by promoting laxation, decreasing transit time, and binding substances such as bile acids and carcinogens. However, evidence to date is insufficient to determine if decreased colon cancer risk is a beneficial effect of this type of fiber.

Selective prebiotic fiber sources, such as inulin, resistant starches, and some oligosaccharides, act as selective substrate for bacteria that produce specific short-chain fatty acids (SCFA) and can lower the intestinal pH. The SCFA butyrate has been shown to increase apoptosis in human colonic tumor cell lines. Apoptosis is a mechanism where excess or redundant cells are removed during development and restricted tissue size is maintained. The apoptosis process is thus an innate cellular defense against carcinogenesis. Evidence suggests that increasing the numbers of Bifidobacteria in the colon and reducing intestinal pH has a direct impact on carcinogenesis in the large intestine. Possible mechanisms for the anticarcinogenic and antitumorigenic effect of highly fermentable fibers are not completely understood and require further research. However, it is likely that some or all are involved in a metabolic chain reaction for the inhibitory effect to occur. The primary mechanisms involved with these effects are proposed to be: a reduction in the production of carcinogenic substances by decreasing the amount of pathogenic bacteria in the colon and/or lowering the colonic pH to affect pH-dependent enzymatic reactions; for example, secondary bile acid formation and/or reducing the amount of carcinogenic substances available to colonic mucosa by adsorption of the substances to the cell wall of the microbiota, by speeding up the intestinal transit time and by increasing colonic contents and thus diluting all components; and/or exerting inhibiting effects on initiation and promotionstages in colon cancer formation in which SCFA, particularly butyric acid, may play a key role .

Mineral bioavailability

Certain fiber sources from fruits and vegetables that have cation exchange capacity from unmethylated galacturonic acid residues and phytic acid from cereal fibers, have been found to depress the absorption and retention of several minerals. However, certain highly fermentable fibers have resulted in improved metabolic absorption of certain minerals, such as calcium, magnesium, and iron, even when phytic acid is present at lower concentrations. These compounds include pectin, various gums, resistant starches, cellulose, certain oligosaccharides like soy and fructo oligosaccharides, inulin, lactulose, and related sugars. Mineral absorption has generally been accepted as stemming from diffusion in the small intestine. However, studies now indicate that highly fermentable fibers, such as inulin and fructo oligosaccharides, also promote mineral absorption in the colon. Through their fermentation by colonic microbiota and subsequent SCFA production, these fi ber components stimulate the proliferation of epithelial cells in the cecocolon and reduce the luminal pH. Al salts, especially calcium, magnesium, and iron, in the luminal content and increase their diffusive absorption via the paracellular route. In particular, the accumulation of calcium phosphate in the large intestine and the solubilization of minerals by SCFA are likely to play an essential role in the enhanced mineral absorption in the colon. Also, a recent study has demonstrated that fructo oligosaccharides (inulin) stimulate the transcellular route of calcium absorption in the large intestine, as indicated by increased concentrations of calbindin-D9k, a calcium binding protein that plays an important role in intestinal calcium transport .

Recommendations for dietary fiber intake

Current recommendations for dietary fiber intake are related to age, gender, and energy intake, and the general recommendation for adequate intake (AI) is 14 g/1000 kcal. This AI includes nonstarch polysaccharides, analogous carbohydrates (e.g., resistant starches), lignin, and associated substances. Using the energy guideline of 2000 kcal/day for women and 2600 kcal/day for men, the recommended daily dietary fiber intake is 28 g/day for adult women and 36 g/day for adult men.

Conclusion

In conclusion, dietary fibers have emerged as versatile nutraceuticals with multiple applications in various disease conditions. Their unique properties and physiological effects make them valuable in promoting overall health and managing specific ailments. The consumption of dietary fibers has been linked to a range of benefits, including improved digestion, weight management, cardiovascular health, and glucose control. In conditions such as obesity, diabetes, and cardiovascular diseases, dietary fibers have shown promising results in reducing risk factors and improving outcomes. Furthermore, the ability of dietary fibers to modulate the gut microbiota and promote a healthy gut environment highlights their potential in managing gastrointestinal disorders, such as irritable bowel syndrome and inflammatory bowel disease. Their prebiotic properties foster the growth of beneficial bacteria, leading to enhanced immune function and reduced inflammation.

In addition to their effects on metabolic and gastrointestinal health, dietary fibers have also demonstrated potential in preventing certain types of cancer, including colorectal cancer. Their ability to bind toxins and carcinogens, as well as promote bowel regularity, contributes to their protective role against cancer development. Moreover, dietary fibers can play a crucial role in managing chronic diseases, including hypertension and hypercholesterolemia. By reducing cholesterol absorption, promoting bile acid excretion, and improving blood pressure regulation, they contribute to maintaining cardiovascular health and reducing the risk of related complications.

Overall, the diverse uses of dietary fibers as nutraceuticals in different disease conditions underscore their significance in preventive healthcare and the management of chronic ailments. However, further research is needed to explore optimal dosage, specific fiber types, and their individual effects on various disease states. As our understanding of the intricate relationship between dietary fibers and human health continues to evolve, incorporating them into therapeutic strategies holds immense potential in improving outcomes and enhancing overall well-being.

References

1. AACC. 2010. Adopts oat bran defi nition. [online], http://www.aaccnet.org/news/pdfs/ OatBran.pdf [accessed: 12 October 2010].
2. American Heart Association. 2008. Cardiovascular disease statistics. [online], www.americanheart.org/presenter. jhtml?identifi er=4478 [accessed: 6 May 2008].
3. Anderson J.W., 2008. Dietary fi ber and associated phytochemicals in prevention and reversal of diabetes. In: Nutraceuticals, glycemic health and type 2 diabetes. Eds V.K. Pasupuleti, J.W. Anderson. Blackwell Publ. Profes. Ames, Iowa, 111-142.
4. Andersson M., Ellegard L., Andersson H., 2002. Oat bran stimulates bile acid synthesis within 8 h as measured by 7 alpha-hydroxy-4-cholesten-3-one. Am. J. Clin. Nutr. 76, 1111-1116.
5. Baer D.J., Rumpler W.V., Miles C.W., Fahey G.C., 1997. Dietary fi ber decreases the metabolizable energy content and nutrient digestibility of mixed diets fed to humans. J. Nutri. Rev. 127, 579-586
6. Codex Alimentarius Commission. 2010. [online], http://www.codexalimentarius. net/download/standards/34/CXG _002e.pdf [accessed: 12 October 2010]
7. Du H.D., Daphne van der A., Boshuizen H.C., Forouhi N.G., Wareham N.J., Halkjaer J., Tjonneland A., Overvad K., Jakobsen M.U., Boeing H., 2010. Dietary fi ber and subsequent changes in body weight and waist circumference in European men and women. Am. J. Clin. Nutr. Rev. 91, 329-336.
8. Escrig A.J., Muniz F.J.S., 2000. Dietary fi bre from edible seaweeds: chemical structure, physicochemical properties

and effects on cholesterol metabolism. Nutr. Rev. 20, 585-598

9. James M.L., Mark D.H., 2010. Effects of dietary fi ber and its components on metabolic health. Nutrients 2 (12), 1266-1289

10. Jensen M.K., Koh-Banerjee P., Hu F.B., Franz M., Sampson L., Gronbaek M., Rimm E.B., 2004. Intakes of whole grains, bran, and germ and the risk of coronary heart disease in men. Am. J. Clin. Nutri. Rev. 80, 1492-1499

11. Jones J., 2000. Update on defi ning dietary fi ber. Cereal Foods World 45, 219-220.

12. Koh-Banerjee P., Franz M.V., Sampson L., Liu S.M., Jacobs D.R., Spiegelman D., Willett W., Rimm E., 2004. Changes in whole-grain, bran, and cereal fi ber consumption in relation to 8-y weight gain among men. Am. J. Clin. Nutri. Rev. 80, 1237-1245.

13. Kris-Etherton P.M., Etherton T.D., Carlson J., Gardner C., 2002. Recent discoveries in inclusive food-based approaches and dietary patterns for reduction in risk for cardiovascular disease. Curr. Opin. Lipidol. 13, 397-407.

14. Merchant A.T., Hu F.B., Spiegelman D., Willett W.C., Rimm E.B., Ascherio A., 2003. Dietary fi ber reduces peripheral arterial disease risk in men. J. Nutri. Rev. 133, 3658-3663

15. Rowland I.R., Rumney C.J., Coutts J.T., Lievense L.C., 1998. Effect of Bifi dobacterium longum and inulin on gut bacterial metabolism and carcinogen-induced aberrant crypt foci in rats. Carcinogenesis 19, 281-285

16. Rumney C., Rowland I.R., 1995. Nondigestible oligosaccharides-potential anti-cancer agents. BNF Nutri. Bull. 20, 194-203.

17. Stampfer M.J., Hu F.B., Manson J.E., Rimm E.B., Willett W.C., 2000. Primary prevention of coronary heart

disease in women through diet and lifestyle. New Eng. J. Med. 343, 16-22.

18. Theuwissen E., Mensink R.P., 2008. Water-soluble dietary fi bers and cardiovascular disease. Phys. Behav. 94, 285-292

19. Tungland B.C., Meyer D., 2006. Nondigestible oligo- and polysaccharides (dietary fi ber): Their physiology and role in human health and food. Compr. Rev. Food Sci. Food Saf. 20, 97-98

20. USDA. 2005. US Department of Agriculture. US Department of Health and Human Services. Dietary Guidelines for Americans. USDA, Washington, DC.

21. Witwer R.S., 2008. Natural resistant starch in glycemic management: from physiological mechanisms to consumer communications. In: Nutraceuticals, glycemic health and Type 2 diabetes. Eds V.K. Pasupuleti, J.W. Anderson. Blackwell Publ. Profes. Ames, Iowa, 401-438.

22. Wong J.M., Jenkins D.J., 2007. Carbohydrate digestibility and metabolic effects. J. Nutr. Rev. 137, 2539-2546

Chapter- 8
Protein Hydrolysates as Nutraceuticals

Introduction

In recent years, there has been a growing interest in the potential health benefits of protein hydrolysates as nutraceuticals. Nutraceuticals are bioactive compounds derived from food sources, with demonstrated physiological benefits beyond their basic nutritional value. Proteins, the building blocks of life, play critical roles in various biological processes, serving as enzymes, hormones, and transporters, and contributing to tissue repair and growth. While intact proteins are vital for meeting our daily protein needs, advances in food science and biotechnology have unlocked the potential of protein hydrolysates as a novel and efficient approach to deliver bioactive peptides, which are short sequences of amino acids derived from protein digestion. These bioactive peptides exhibit specific physiological effects, giving rise to their role as nutraceuticals with potential health-promoting properties. Protein hydrolysates are obtained by breaking down larger proteins into smaller peptides through enzymatic, chemical, or microbial processes. This chapter explores the emerging research on protein hydrolysates and their potential as nutraceuticals in promoting human health and wellness.

Production and Types of Protein Hydrolysates :

1) **Enzymatic Hydrolysis** : Enzymatic hydrolysis is one of the most common methods used to produce protein hydrolysates. It involves the use of enzymes to break down larger protein molecules into smaller peptides. Proteases, such as trypsin, papain, and bromelain, are commonly used enzymes in this process. Enzymatic hydrolysis offers control over the degree of hydrolysis, allowing manufacturers to

obtain specific peptide profiles with desired bioactive properties.

2) **Chemical Hydrolysis :** Chemical hydrolysis involves the use of acids or alkaline solutions to break down proteins into peptides. While this method is more cost-effective, it often results in a less defined peptide profile compared to enzymatic hydrolysis. Additionally, chemical hydrolysis can lead to the formation of undesirable by-products and potential safety concerns.

3) **Microbial Hydrolysis :** Microbial hydrolysis relies on the action of microorganisms, such as bacteria or yeast, to break down proteins into peptides. This method can be more sustainable and environmentally friendly compared to chemical processes. However, controlling the specificity of peptide formation can be more challenging with microbial hydrolysis.

Sources of Proteins for Hydrolysate Production : Protein hydrolysates can be derived from various sources, such as animal proteins (e.g., whey, casein, collagen) and plant proteins (e.g., soy, pea, rice). Different sources yield protein hydrolysates with varying peptide profiles, which can influence their bioactivity and potential health benefits.

Bioactive Peptides in Protein Hydrolysates :

▪ **Bioactive Peptides and Health Benefits**: Bioactive peptides are short chains of amino acids derived from proteins that have specific physiological effects beyond their basic nutritional value. In protein hydrolysates, these peptides can exhibit a wide range of health benefits due to their interactions with specific biological targets in the body.

▪ **Antioxidant Peptides**: Antioxidant peptides scavenge free radicals and reduce oxidative stress, potentially protecting cells from damage. These peptides have been studied for their role in reducing the risk of chronic diseases associated with oxidative damage, such as cardiovascular disease and certain cancers.

▪ **Antihypertensive Peptides** : Antihypertensive peptides have the ability to lower blood pressure by inhibiting enzymes that contribute to hypertension. Their potential role in managing hypertension makes them a focus of research for cardiovascular health.

▪ **Immunomodulatory Peptides**: Immunomodulatory peptides can modulate the immune system, either by enhancing or suppressing immune responses. They are of interest in supporting immune function and may have implications in autoimmune conditions and infectious diseases.

▪ **Anti-inflammatory Peptides** : Anti-inflammatory peptides can help reduce inflammation in the body by inhibiting pro-inflammatory pathways. Chronic inflammation is associated with various health conditions, and anti-inflammatory peptides may have therapeutic potential in managing inflammatory disorders.

▪ **Antimicrobial Peptides** : Antimicrobial peptides have antimicrobial properties, meaning they can kill or inhibit the growth of microorganisms such as bacteria, fungi, and viruses. They are being explored as potential alternatives to conventional antimicrobial agents to combat antimicrobial resistance.

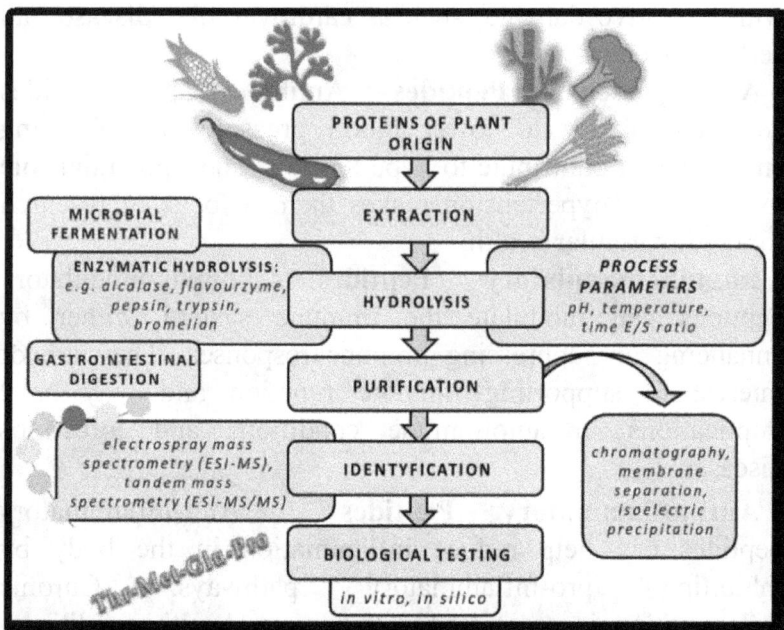

Figure 1: Diagrammatic representation of bioactive peptide preparation from plant origin, (Czelej et al.,2022)

Health Benefits of Protein Hydrolysates as Nutraceuticals

❖ **Muscle Health and Exercise Recovery :** Protein hydrolysates, particularly those rich in branched-chain amino acids, are commonly used in sports nutrition for muscle recovery and repair after intense exercise. They can aid in promoting muscle protein synthesis and reducing muscle protein breakdown.

❖ **Weight Management and Satiety :** Certain protein hydrolysates have been shown to enhance satiety, leading to reduced food intake and potentially supporting weight management efforts.

❖ **Cardiovascular Health :** The antihypertensive and antioxidant properties of some protein hydrolysates make them potential candidates for promoting cardiovascular health by managing blood pressure and reducing oxidative stress.

❖ **Gut Health and Digestive Enzymes** : Bioactive peptides in protein hydrolysates can influence gut health by promoting the growth of beneficial gut bacteria and improving digestive enzyme activity.

❖ **Cognitive Function and Brain Health** : Peptides with neuroprotective properties found in protein hydrolysates have been studied for their potential in supporting cognitive function and brain health, with implications in age-related cognitive decline and neurodegenerative diseases.

❖ **Bone Health** : Some protein hydrolysates may contain peptides that support bone health by enhancing calcium absorption and promoting bone mineralization.

❖ **Skin Health** : Bioactive peptides in protein hydrolysates may have benefits for skin health, including promoting collagen synthesis and providing antioxidant support against skin aging

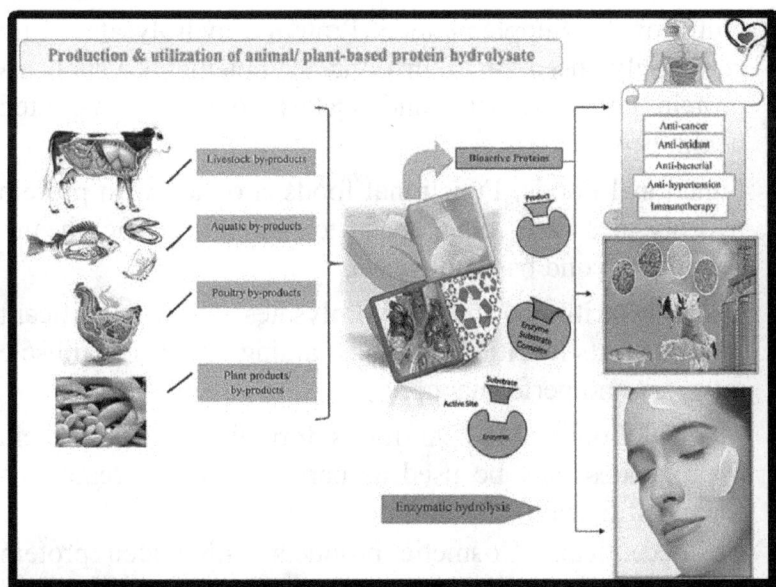

Figure 2 : Pictorial representation of production and utilization of animal/plant based hydrolysates (Etemadian et al., 2021)

Absorption, Bioavailability, and Safety

• **Absorption of Protein Hydrolysates** : The degree of hydrolysis and the size of the peptides influence their absorption in the digestive tract. Smaller peptides are generally better absorbed and have higher bioavailability.

• **Bioavailability of Bioactive Peptides** : The bioavailability of bioactive peptides depends on various factors, such as their structure, interaction with other food components, and potential degradation by digestive enzymes.

• **Safety Considerations and Allergenicity** : While protein hydrolysates can offer numerous health benefits, potential allergenicity and the presence of undesirable by-products are critical safety considerations in their use.

Applications of Protein Hydrolysates in Nutraceutical Products :

• Nutritional Supplements: Protein hydrolysates are commonly used in nutritional supplements, such as protein powders, bars, and shakes, to provide targeted health benefits.

• Functional Foods: Functional foods enriched with protein hydrolysates are developed to offer specific health benefits beyond basic nutrition.

• Sports Nutrition: Protein hydrolysates play a significant role in sports nutrition products, aiding athletes in muscle recovery and performance.

• Medical Foods: Medical foods formulated with protein hydrolysates may be used as part of medical treatments for specific health conditions.

• Cosmeceuticals: Cosmetic products with added protein hydrolysates are gaining popularity due to their potential benefits for skin health and anti-aging effects.

Future Perspectives and Challenges

- Regulatory Frameworks and Labeling: Developing appropriate regulatory frameworks and clear labeling guidelines is essential for the safe and effective use of protein hydrolysates as nutraceuticals.

- Personalized Nutrition and Precision Medicine: Advancements in understanding individual genetic variations and responses to nutrients may lead to personalized approaches in utilizing protein hydrolysates for optimal health.

- Sustainability and Environmental Impact: The sustainability of protein sources and the environmental impact of hydrolysate production need to be considered in the future development of nutraceutical products.

- Technological Advances in Hydrolysate Production: Continued research in enzymatic and microbial hydrolysis processes could lead to more efficient and targeted production of bioactive peptides.

Conclusion :

In conclusion, the exploration of protein hydrolysates as nutraceuticals has opened a fascinating realm in the domain of functional foods and health-promoting compounds. The journey through this chapter has provided a comprehensive understanding of the production methods, types, and health benefits of protein hydrolysates, shedding light on their potential as powerful bioactive agents.

The production of protein hydrolysates using enzymatic, chemical, and microbial methods offers versatility in tailoring the composition of bioactive peptides. Enzymatic hydrolysis, in particular, allows for precise control over peptide profiles, enabling the development of targeted nutraceutical products with specific health benefits. However, it is essential to strike a balance between cost-effectiveness and purity while ensuring the safety and

97

allergenicity of the final product.

Bioactive peptides found in protein hydrolysates have shown remarkable potential in supporting diverse aspects of human health. Antioxidant peptides combat oxidative stress, offering protection against chronic diseases, while antihypertensive peptides contribute to cardiovascular health by managing blood pressure. Immunomodulatory and anti-inflammatory peptides showcase their significance in bolstering the immune system and mitigating inflammatory responses, respectively. The antimicrobial properties of certain peptides offer potential alternatives in the fight against microbial infections.

The health benefits of protein hydrolysates extend beyond the cardiovascular and immune systems. Their role in supporting muscle health and exercise recovery makes them invaluable in sports nutrition, aiding athletes and fitness enthusiasts in their pursuit of peak performance. Additionally, the potential of protein hydrolysates in weight management, gut health, cognitive function, bone health, and skin health underscores their multifaceted nature as nutraceuticals.

Ensuring the optimal absorption and bioavailability of bioactive peptides is essential to fully harness the potential of protein hydrolysates. Further research in this area will lead to improved formulations and enhanced efficacy of nutraceutical products, ultimately benefiting consumers seeking personalized nutrition approaches.

While the future of protein hydrolysates as nutraceuticals appears promising, several challenges must be addressed. Regulatory frameworks and labeling guidelines need to be developed to ensure the safe and responsible use of these functional ingredients. Consumer education and awareness play a pivotal role in promoting the acceptance and integration of protein hydrolysates into everyday diets.

As scientific knowledge continues to advance, new opportunities and applications for protein hydrolysates may emerge. The intersection of personalized nutrition and precision medicine holds promise in tailoring nutraceutical products to individual needs and genetic predispositions. Moreover, the sustainability and environmental impact of protein sources and hydrolysate production warrant careful consideration to maintain ecological balance and responsible resource utilization.

In summary, the potential of protein hydrolysates as nutraceuticals remains an exciting frontier, offering a myriad of health benefits and opportunities for personalized well-being. The continued collaboration among researchers, manufacturers, regulatory bodies, and consumers will play a pivotal role in unlocking the full potential of protein hydrolysates as vital tools for enhancing human health and contributing to a future of holistic and personalized nutrition. With each step forward, we embark on an inspiring journey towards improved health and wellness through the transformative power of protein hydrolysates as nutraceuticals.

References
1. Czelej, M., Garbacz, K., Czernecki, T., Wawrzykowski, J., & Waśko, A. (2022). Protein hydrolysates derived from animals and plants—a review of production methods and antioxidant activity. *Foods*, *11*(13), 1953.
2. Etemadian, Y., Ghaemi, V., Shaviklo, A. R., Pourashouri, P., Mahoonak, A. R. S., & Rafipour, F. (2021). Development of animal/plant-based protein hydrolysate and its application in food, feed and nutraceutical industries: State of the art. *Journal of Cleaner Production*, *278*, 123219.

3. Fuentes-Alventosa, J. M., Rodríguez-Gutiérrez, G., & Jaramillo-Carmona, S. (2019). Nutraceutical potential of protein hydrolysates derived from the tuna canning industry. Journal of Aquatic Food Product Technology, 28(4), 403-412. doi:10.1080/10498850.2018.1532556

4. Hayes, M., & Mora, L. (2019). Bioactive peptides: Significance, bioaccessibility, and potential uses. Nutrients, 11(11), 2805. doi:10.3390/nu11112805

5. Hernández-Ledesma, B., & Recio, I. (2008). Antioxidant and other biological activities of milk proteins and peptides. Current Pharmaceutical Design, 14(8), 829-843. doi:10.2174/138161208784746203

6. Jäger, R., Kerksick, C. M., Campbell, B. I., Cribb, P. J., Wells, S. D., Skwiat, T. M., . . . Antonio, J. (2017). International Society of Sports Nutrition position stand: Protein and exercise. Journal of the International Society of Sports Nutrition, 14(1), 20. doi:10.1186/s12970-017-0177-8

7. Kitts, D. D., & Weiler, K. (2003). Bioactive proteins and peptides from food sources. Applications of bioprocesses used in isolation and recovery. Current Pharmaceutical Design, 9(16), 1309-1323. doi:10.2174/1381612033454897

8. Li, G. H., Le, G. W., Shi, Y. H., Shrestha, S., & Ang, L. E. (2019). Identification and purification of a novel antioxidant peptide from chickpea (Cicer arietinum L.) protein hydrolysates. Food Chemistry, 277, 71-78. doi:10.1016/j.foodchem.2018.10.145

9. Martínez-Maqueda, D., Miralles, B., Recio, I., & Hernández-Ledesma, B. (2012). Antihypertensive peptides from food proteins: A review. Food & Function, 3(4), 350-361. doi:10.1039/c2fo10294d

10. Mine, Y. (2019). Recent advances in the understanding of egg bioactive peptides. Journal of Agricultural and

Food Chemistry, 67(31), 8597-8601. doi:10.1021/acs.jafc.9b03757
11. Wu, H., & He, H. L. (2018). Protein hydrolysates and biopeptides: Production, biological activities, and applications in foods and health benefits. Food & Nutrition Research, 62, 1368. doi:10.29219/fnr.v62.1368
12. Xu, Y., Su, Y., & Wang, T. (2018). Chemical and enzymatic hydrolysis in the preparation of bioactive peptides from casein. Journal of Dairy Science, 101(4), 2305-2317. doi:10.3168/jds.2017-13234

Chapter- 9

Nutraceutical properties of Millets

Introduction

Nutraceuticals extracted from millets represent an intriguing fusion of nutrition and medicine. Millets, a cluster of tiny-seed grasses, have gained attention for being rich in nutrients and bioactive elements like antioxidants, phenolic compounds, fibers, vitamins, and minerals. Sorghum, finger millet, pearl millet, among others, are celebrated for their nutritional prowess and adaptability to various climates.

These nutraceuticals from millets offer a spectrum of health benefits, from managing diabetes and obesity to enhancing heart health and aiding digestion, thanks to their diverse bioactive compounds. The marriage of ancient knowledge with modern scientific discoveries highlights millets' potential as functional foods and nutraceutical sources. They're not just sustenance but a reservoir of medicinal compounds with promising health properties.

Ongoing research delves deeper into millets, uncovering more bioactive components and inspiring the creation of innovative nutraceutical products. Exploring millets for nutraceutical purposes aligns with the trend toward natural, whole-food remedies and emphasizes the value of traditional food sources in addressing modern health concerns.

Phenolic Compounds

The diverse range of phenolic compounds discovered in millets - from phenolic acids to flavonoids and lignans - signifies their potential as robust antioxidants and agents for promoting health. Research has identified significant variations in polyphenol levels across different millet varieties, with higher concentrations observed in brown varieties compared to white ones.Extracted bound polyphenols from various millet types display remarkable antioxidant properties, capable of combating oxidative stress linked to conditions such as cancer and cardiovascular diseases. These compounds offer a spectrum of health benefits, including anti-obesity, anti-diabetic, antimicrobial, and antiviral effects.

The mechanism driving the antioxidant action of phenolic compounds lies in their ability to donate hydrogen atoms to free radicals, neutralizing their reactivity. Their hydroxyl groups in the benzene rings play a crucial role in forming stabilized phenoxyl radicals. Additionally, phenolic compounds have shown inhibitory effects on various digestive enzymes like amylase, glucosidase, pepsin, trypsin, and lipases. This inhibition is particularly relevant in managing type 2 diabetes by reducing post-meal hyper-glycemia, resembling the action of medications like acarbose, miglitol, and voglibose, contributing to blood glucose regulation.The combined action and synergy among different phenolic compounds amplify their health benefits, correlating their presence in diets with a lowered risk of chronic diseases. This emphasizes their potential in preventive healthcare strategies.

In summary, the concentration of phenolic compounds in millets, especially the bound polyphenols, emphasizes their significance as a valuable source of health-enhancing antioxidants. Their multifaceted properties hold immense potential in preventing and managing diseases, notably in conditions like diabetes and oxidative stress-related ailments.

Phenolic Acids

Phenolic acids, characterized by a benzene ring and a carboxylic acid function, fall into two main groups: hydroxybenzoic acid and hydroxycinnamic acid derivatives. Hydroxybenzoic acid derivatives, like hydroxybenzoic, protocatechuic, vanillic, syringic, and gallic acids, often exist in bound forms within complex structures such as lignins and hydrolyzable tannins. On the flip side, hydroxycinnamic acid derivatives, such as p-coumaric, caffeic, ferulic, and sinapic acids, are commonly bound to cell wall components like cellulose, lignin, and proteins through ester bonds.

Within finger millet grains, several prominent phenolic acids include ferulic acid, vanillic acid, caffeic acid, syringic acid, and p-coumaric acid. Ferulic acid, notably abundant in the aleurone, pericarp, and embryo cell walls of various grains, is present in minimal quantities within the starchy endosperm. Its significance lies notably in its role as a key phenolic acid in finger millet grains.

Flavonoids

Flavonoids, a varied group of compounds derived from plants, feature a 15-carbon structure comprising two phenyl rings and a heterocyclic ring. Originating from phenylalanine, these pigments showcase a fundamental C6-C3-C6 structure, embodying various polyphenolic compounds like anthocyanins, flavonols, flavanols, and isoflavones. Typically, flavonoids are glycosides, except for flavanols, which commonly form condensed tannins.

Two primary forms of tannins exist in flavonoids: condensed and hydrolyzable tannins. Condensed tannins are often polymers of flavan-3-ols (catechins) or flavan-3,4-diols (leucoanthocyanidins), while hydrolyzable tannins are esters of glucose or polyhydric alcohols with gallic acid (gallotannins) or hexahydrodiphenic acid (ellagitannins). Compounds like catechin, quercetin, anthocyanins, and tannins offer notable health benefits owing to their radical-scavenging abilities.

The antioxidant potency of flavonoids relies on the arrangement and quantity of hydroxyl groups within their structure, combined with the presence of electron-donating and electron-withdrawing groups. Studies comparing antioxidant activity have highlighted that whole grains possess similar antioxidant potential per serving as fruits and vegetables.

Millets, especially finger millet, are recognized as sources of specific flavones. For example, finger millet leaves contain eight types of flavones: vitexin, isovitexin, saponarin, violanthin, orientin, isoorientin, lucenin-1, and tricin. Different millet types such as pearl millet, Japanese barnyard millet, and fonio have been found to contain various flavones, each with distinct compositions.

Finger millet notably stands out as the sole millet containing condensed tannins, with higher content observed in brown varieties compared to white ones. However, detailed structural characterizations of millet proanthocyanidins remain a gap in current research.

In essence, flavonoids discovered in millets comprise a diverse range of compounds boasting significant antioxidant properties, showcasing their potential health advantages. This emphasizes the importance of incorporating these grains into a well-rounded diet rich in phytochemicals.

Phytic Acid

Phytic acid, also known as myoinositol 1,2,3,4,5,6 hexakis-dihydrogen phosphate, is typically present in foods at concentrations ranging from 0.1 to 6.0%. Studies have identified its primary location in the bran of cereal grains or within the cotyledons of oilseeds and legumes, often enclosed within protein bodies.

Research conducted by Reddy et al. in 1982 delineated the distribution of phytic acid across different parts of grains. Lorenz's study reported phytate content in various common millet varieties, ranging from 170 to 470 mg/100 g in whole grain. Moreover, processes like dehulling have been observed to reduce phytate content. For example, dehulling resulted in reductions of 27–53% in phytate content across various millet varieties: 12% in common millet, 39% in little millet, 25% in kodo millet, and 23% in barnyard millet.

Carotenoid and Tocopherols

Carotenoids, a group encompassing over 600 pigments found in various foods, are well-known for their role as provitamin-A compounds. Beyond their provitamin-A activity, they function as antioxidants, playing a crucial role in safeguarding against a range of diseases. Structurally, carotenoids consist of isoprenoid units forming a lengthy polyene chain with 3 to 15 conjugated double bonds. The placement of these double bonds determines their absorption spectrum. Carotenes are cyclized products, while xanthophylls result from oxygen addition, with potential modifications through isomerization, elongation, or degradation.

Recent research by Asharani et al. unveiled the total carotenoid content in edible millet flour, ranging from 78 to 366 μg/100 g. Finger, little, foxtail, and proso millets displayed average carotenoid values of 199 μg/100 g, 78 μg/100 g, 173 μg/100 g, and 366 μg/100 g, respectively. While millet's carotenoid content is comparable to wheat (150–200 μg/100 g) and sorghum (180–230 μg/100 g), it notably falls short of maize (1800–5500 μg/100 g) and its variations (2400-3200 μg/100 g).

Vitamin E, a fat-soluble compound existing in eight different molecules, shares a chromanol ring and a 12-carbon aliphatic side chain. This family comprises four saturated tocopherols and four tocotrienols, the latter featuring three double bonds. Variations within tocopherols and tocotrienols—alpha, beta, gamma, and delta—are attributed to the number of methyl groups in the chain. High-performance liquid chromatography (HPLC) analysis of millets indicated higher levels of γ- and α-tocopherols and lower levels of tocotrienols. Finger and proso millet varieties exhibited greater total tocopherol content (3.6–4.0 mg/100 g) compared to foxtail and little millet varieties (~1.3 mg/100 g). Vitamin E acts as an antioxidant and anti-inflammatory agent, reduces superoxide production in mitochondria, and possesses anti-atherosclerotic properties.

Phytosterols

Phytosterols, similar in ring structure to cholesterol, are essential components in plant cells. Their resemblance to cholesterol allows them to significantly decrease serum cholesterol levels by regulating the absorption rates of both dietary and internally produced cholesterol.

Phytosterol esters have shown the potential to lower LDL cholesterol levels in blood serum by up to 14%, without affecting HDL levels. Regular consumption of phytosterols can reduce the risk of heart diseases by as much as 40%, although the effectiveness may vary depending on age and other contributing factors. However, it's important to note that while phytosterols offer these cholesterol-lowering benefits, their presence can inhibit the absorption of alpha and beta-carotene, as well as Vitamin E.

The absorption of phytosterols can be influenced by processes like etherification, emulsification, and solubilization, which can negatively impact their bioavailability. Finger millet has been reported to contain a phytosterol content of 0.149% based on seed weight, while other millets typically contain only minimal amounts. In comparison, sorghum and corn have reported phytosterol contents of 0.5 mg/g and 0.9 mg/g, respectively.

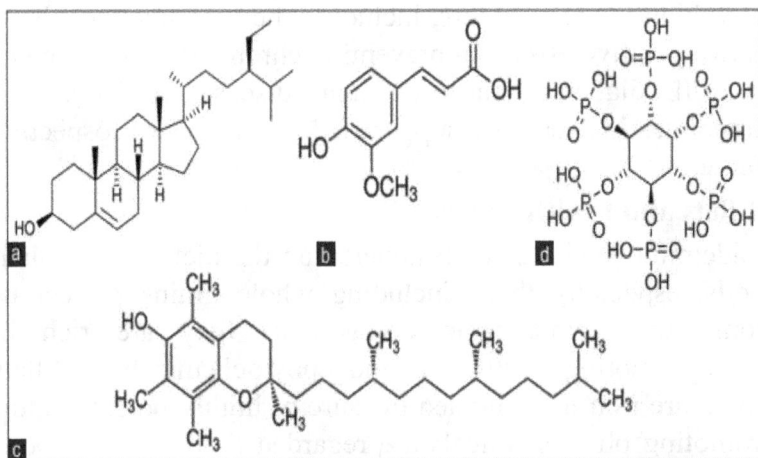

Figure 1: Structure of molecules (a) Phytosterols (b) Ferulic acid (c) Alpha-tocopherol (d) Phytic acid

107

Arabinoxylans

Arabinoxylans, a type of hemicellulose present in plant cell walls, are found in both primary and secondary cell walls. They consist of a chain of 1,4-linked xylose with 2,3-linked arabinose residues, functioning as dietary fibers due to their indigestible nature. Fibers like arabinoxylans add bulk to the diet and contribute positively to cholesterol regulation.

The content of xylooligosaccharides in finger millet bran is estimated at 15.60%, while wheat bran contains roughly 40%, and corn bran about 9.33%. Arabinoxylans undergo enzymatic hydrolysis, generating arabinoxylan-oligosaccharides (AXOS), comprising arabinoxy-looligosaccharides and xylooligosaccharides (XOS). This breakdown occurs during cereal processing, bread and beer production, and within the colon through bacterial fermentation.

Studies have highlighted that compounds like AXOS and XOS exhibit a prebiotic effect in the human and animal colon by selectively stimulating beneficial intestinal microbiota. Dietary fibers, including these compounds, have shown positive effects in preventing chronic diseases such as type II diabetes, cardiovascular diseases (CVD), and gastrointestinal cancer, supported by extensive prospective studies.

Millets and health effects

Epidemiological studies conducted on the diets rich in plant foods, especially those including whole grains protect us from non-communicable diseases as they are rich in healthpromoting nutrients and phytochemicals. Millets which are rich in its hidden treasure of highly potent health-promoting phytochemicals are regarded as functional foods (Figure 2).

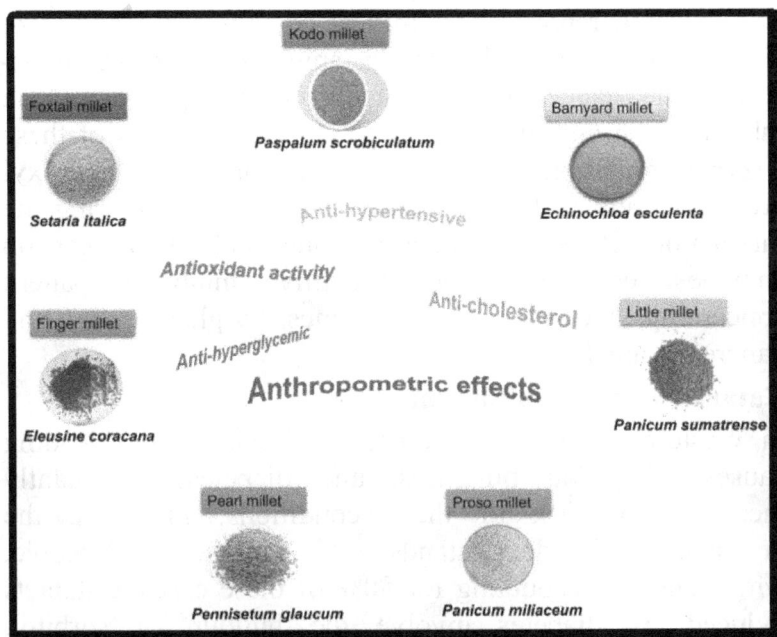

Figure 2 : Different types of millets and its therapeutic effects

Diabetes

Epidemiological research indicates a lower occurrence of diabetes among populations consuming millets. In a study by Kumari and Sumathi (2002), the impact of consuming finger millet on non-insulin-dependent diabetes mellitus (NIDDM) was investigated. It was discovered that the glycemic index of finger millet was lower compared to rice and wheat, likely due to the presence of polyphenols in whole finger millet flour. These polyphenols are recognized for reducing starch digestibility and absorption. Finger millet polyphenols (FMP) were extracted using acidified methanol and then assessed for their ability to hinder the activities of porcine pancreatic α-amylase and rat intestinal α-glucosidase. This suggests substantial potential for these phenolics in managing hyperglycemia.

Tadera et al. reported that millets contain compounds like naringenin, kaempferol, luteolin, apigenin, (+)-catechin/(-)-epicatechin, daidzein, and epigallocatechin gallate, which inhibit starch digestive enzymes. The effectiveness of these enzyme inhibitions is linked to the number of hydroxyl groups present in flavonoids. Kinetic studies exploring the interaction between seed coat phenolics and starch digestion enzymes revealed a non-competitive inhibition pattern concerning the two key enzymes, α-glucosidase and pancreatic amylase.

Cataractogenesis Inhibition

In Western countries, retinopathy and cataracts are leading causes of global blindness, and diabetes significantly increases the risk of these conditions. In India, the prevalence of blindness stands at 15 cases per 1000 people, with cataracts accounting for 80% of these cases. Cataracts induced by diabetes involve the buildup of sorbitol, facilitated by the enzyme aldose reductase (AR). The process of non-enzymatic glycation, where glucose binds to protein molecules, is a key initiator of sugar-induced cataracts mediated by aldose reductase during diabetes.

Chethan et al. explored the potential of Finger Millet Polyphenols (FMP) to inhibit aldose reductase (AR), emphasizing their role as potential antioxidants and antidiabetic agents. Various phenolic components present in FMP, such as gallic acid, protocatechuic acid, p-hydroxybenzoic acid, p-coumaric acid, vanillic acid, syringic acid, ferulic acid, trans-cinnamic acid, and quercetin, demonstrated effective inhibition of cataracts in the eye lens. Detailed analysis of these phenolics revealed that the presence of a hydroxyl group at the 4th position played a critical role in aldose reductase inhibition. Furthermore, the presence of an adjacent O-methyl group to the –OH group in these phenolics was observed to impact the denaturation of aldose reductase activity.

Wound Healing and Nerve Growth Factor (NGF) Production

Rajasekaran et al. conducted a study examining the effects of incorporating finger millet into the diets of early diabetic rats and its influence on skin antioxidants, nerve growth factor (NGF) production, and wound healing. The research involved feeding hyperglycemic rats a diet containing 50 grams of finger millet per 100 grams. Full-thickness skin wounds were created two weeks after initiating the finger millet diet, and multiple parameters were assessed throughout the healing process.

The study found that wound healing in hyperglycemic rats fed a finger millet diet was expedited, demonstrating an accelerated rate of wound closure. Interestingly, thiobarbituric acid reactive substances (TBARS) levels, indicating increased oxidative stress, were elevated in all wound tissue groups compared to normal skin tissues. However, diabetic rats showed significantly higher TBARS levels in both normal and wounded skin tissues compared to the control group and diabetic rats fed a non-finger millet diet.

Furthermore, impaired NGF production in diabetic rats notably improved with finger millet incorporation into their diet, as confirmed by ELISA and immunocytochemical assessments revealing heightened NGF expression. Histological and electron microscopic evaluations displayed critical signs of healing, including epithelialization, increased collagen synthesis, and activation of fibroblasts and mast cells in animals fed with finger millet.

The study concluded that feeding finger millet for four weeks not only helped regulate glucose levels in diabetic animals but also improved their antioxidant status, expediting the dermal wound healing process. Additionally, there are indications that finger millet consumption may positively affect aortic fragility and elasticity by reducing blood pressure elevation and enhancing vasorelaxation.

Other health beneficial effects:

Millets, owing to their rich fiber content and antioxidants, have showcased the capacity to reduce serum lipid profiles and blood sugar levels. Studies highlight the correlation between increased consumption of proso millet and its derivatives and a lowered risk of chronic conditions, notably elevated serum cholesterol. Shobana et al.'s research suggests that a diet containing 20% millet seed coat matter exhibited hypoglycemic, hypocholesterolemic, nephroprotective, and anticataractogenic properties in diabetic rats induced by streptozotocin. Liver studies also imply that proso millet might act as a preventive food in conditions like hepatic encephalopathy linked to chronic liver failure and injury.

This body of evidence underscores millets' potential in shielding against age-related degenerative diseases. Further exploration of this potential is pivotal, especially considering the prevalence of such ailments in the Indian population. Given that India stands as the largest millet producer, there exists an opportunity to expand into the global market by offering appropriately validated functional foods derived from millets.

Conclusion

Millets play a crucial role in semiarid and tropical regions due to their resilience against pests, short growth cycles, and adaptability to challenging conditions like heat and drought. About 90% of global millet production caters to developing nations, with around two-thirds directly consumed as food, especially among economically disadvantaged populations, serving as a traditional source of health and vigor. Nutritionally, millets match up to popular cereals like rice, wheat, and barley in terms of protein, carbohydrates, and energy content. Their health benefits largely stem from phytochemicals such as polyphenols, tocopherols, phytosterols, dietary fiber, minerals, vitamins, and trace elements. While animal studies strongly support millets' health advantages, human-based evidence, including epidemiology and experiments, is relatively limited. Yet, some epidemiological research suggests that regular millet consumption correlates with reduced risks of chronic illnesses like diabetes, cardiovascular diseases, certain cancers, and overall mortality. Encouraging individuals to incorporate a diverse range of fruits, vegetables, and millet grains into their daily diets seems to be a pragmatic approach for enhancing health and minimizing chronic disease risks.

Despite being among the healthiest choices, millet consumption remains relatively low in developed nations where diet-related chronic diseases prevail. Increasing production while reducing costs through innovative agricultural practices is crucial. Furthermore, refining processing techniques, machinery, and standardizing products is essential. Changing the perception of millets as food primarily for the economically disadvantaged is pivotal. Optimizing processed millet products to deliver maximum benefits to consumers is key. Millets hold the potential to offer a variety of healthy foods and, given their health advantages, warrant extensive promotion to compete with major cereals in terms of utilization.

References

1. Asharani VT, Jayadeep A, Malleshi NG. Natural antioxidants in edible flours of selected small millets. Int J Food Prop 2010;13:41-50.
2. Bailey C J. New approaches to the pharmacotherapy of diabetes (In JC Pickup & G. William (Eds.). Text book of diabetes (Vol. 2, pp. 73.1–73.2).UK: Blackwell Science Ltd 2001.

3. Chandrasekara A, Shahidi F. Content of insoluble bound phenolics in millets and their contribution to antioxidant capacity. J Agric Food Chem 2010;58:6706-14.
4. Chandrasekara A, Shahidi F. Content of insoluble bound phenolics in millets and their contribution to antioxidant capacity. J Agric Food Chem 2010;58:6706-14
5. Chethan S, Dharmesh SM, Malleshi NG. Inhibition of aldose reductase from cataracted eye lenses by finger millet (Eleusine coracana) polyphenols. Bioorg Med Chem 2008;16:10085-90.
6. Chethan S, Dharmesh SM, Malleshi NG. Inhibition of aldose reductase from cataracted eye lenses by finger millet (Eleusine coracana) polyphenols. Bioorg Med Chem 2008;16:10085-90.
7. Chethan S, Malleshi NG. Finger millet polyphenols: Optimization of extraction and the effect of pH on their stability. Food Chem 2007;105:862-70.
8. Chethan S, Sreerama YN, Malleshi NG. Mode of inhibition of finger millet malt amylases by the millet phenolics. Food Chem. 2008;111: p. 187–191
9. de Almeida Rios S, Paes MC, Cardoso WS, Borém A, Teixeira FF. Color of corn grains and carotenoid profile of importance for human health. Am J Plant Sci 2014;5:857-62.
10. Hilu KW, De Wet JM, Seigler D, Flavonoid patterns, Horan FE, Heider MF. A study of sorghum and sorghum starches. Cereal Chem 1978;23:492-503.
11. Jensen MK, Koh-Banerjee P, Hu FB, Franz M, Sampson L, Grønbaek M, et al. Intakes of whole grains, bran, and germ and the risk of coronary heart disease in men. Am J Clin Nutr 2004;80:1492-9.
12. Lakshmi Kumari P, Sumathi S. Effect of consumption of finger millet on hyperglycemia in non-insulin dependent diabetes mellitus (NIDDM) subjects. Plant Foods Hum Nutr 2002;57:205-13.

13. Liu RH. Whole grain phytochemicals and health. J Cereal Sci 2007;46:207-19.
14. Mahadevappa VG, Raina PL. Sterol lipids in finger millet (Eleusine coracana). J Am Oil Chem Soc 1978;55:647-8.
15. Mizutani K, Ikeda K, Kawai Y, Yamori Y. Extract of wine phenolics improves aortic biomechanical properties in strokeprone spontaneously hypertensive rats (SHRSP). J Nutr Sci Vitaminol (Tokyo) 1999;45:95-106.
16. Mori H, Kawabata K, Yoshimi N, Tanaka T, Murakami T, Okada T, et al. Chemopreventive effects of ferulic acid on oral and rice germ on large bowel carcinogenesis. Anticancer Res 1999;19:3775-8.
17. Mozaffarian D, Kumanyika SK, Lemaitre RN, Olson JL, Burke GL, Siscovick DS. Cereal, fruit, and vegetable fiber intake and the risk of cardiovascular disease in elderly individuals. JAMA 2003;289:1659-66.
18. Nishizawa N, Fudamo Y. The elevation of plasma concentration of high density lipoprotein chloesterol in mice fed with protein from proso millet (Panicum miliaceum). Biosci Biotech Biochem 1995;59:333-5.
19. Pietta PG. Flavonoids as antioxidants. J Nat Prod 2000;63:1035-42.
20. Poutanen K, Shepherd R, Shewry PR, Delcour JA, Björck I, van der Kamp JW. Beyond whole grain: The European healthgrain project aims at healthier cereal foods. Cereal Foods World 2008;53:32-5.
21. Rajasekaran NS, Nithya M, Rose C, Chandra TS. The effect of finger millet feeding on the early responses during the process of wound healing in diabetic rats. Biochim Biophys Acta 2004;1689:190-201.
22. Ramachandra G, Virupaksha TK, Shadaksharaswamy M. Relation between tannin levels and in vitro protein digestibility in finger millet (Eleusine coracana Gaertn.). J Agric Food Chem 1977;25:1101-4

23. Rao BR, Nagasampige MH, Ravikiran M. Evaluation of nutraceutical properties of selected small millets. J Pharm Bioallied Sci 2011;3:277-9.
24. Reddy NR, Sathe SK, Salunkhe DK. Phytates in legumes and cereals. Adv Food Res 1982;28:1-92. 45. Harland BF, Oberleas D. Phytate in foods. World Rev Nutr Diet 1987;52:235-59.
25. Reichert RD. The pH-sensitive pigments in pearl millet. Cereal Chem 1979;56:291-4. 41. Watanabe M. Antioxidative phenolic compounds from Japanese barnyard millet (Echinochloa utilis) grains. J Agric Food Chem 1999;47:4500-5.
26. Rohn S, Rawel HM, Kroll J. Inhibitory effects of plant phenols on the activity of selected enzymes. J Agric Food Chem 2002;50:3566-71.
27. Saito N, Sakai H, Suzuki S, Sekihara H, Yajima Y. Effect of an alpha-glucosidase inhibitor (voglibose), in combination with sulphonylureas, on glycaemic control in Type 2 diabetes patients. J Int Med Res 1998;26:219-32.
28. Saleh AS, Zhang Q, Chen J, Shen Q. Millet grains: Nutritional quality and potential health benefits. Compr Rev Food Sci Food Saf 2013;12:281-95
29. Sartelet H, Serghat S, Lobstein A, Ingenbleek Y, Anton R, Petitfrère E, et al. Flavonoids extracted from fonio millet (Digitaria exilis) reveal potent antithyroid properties. Nutrition 1996;12:100-6.
30. Schatzkin A, Mouw T, Park Y, Subar AF, Kipnis V, Hollenbeck A, et al. Dietary fiber and whole-grain consumption in relation to colorectal cancer in the NIH-AARP diet and health study. Am J Clin Nutr 2007;85:1353-60.
31. Shobana S, Harsha MR, Platel K, Srinivasan K, Malleshi NG. Amelioration of hyperglycaemia and its associated complications by finger millet (Eleusine coracana L.)

seed coat matter in streptozotocin-induced diabetic rats. Br J Nutr 2010;104:1787-95

32. Singh V, Moreau RA, Hicks K. Yield and phytosterol composition of oil extracted from grain sorghum and its wetmilled fractions. Cereal Chem 2003;80:126-9.

33. Tadera K, Minami Y, Takamatsu K, Matsuoka T. Inhibition of alpha-glucosidase and alpha-amylase by flavonoids. J Nutr Sci Vitaminol (Tokyo) 2006;52:149-53

34. Toeller M. Alpha-glucosidase inhibitors in diabetes: Efficacy in NIDDM subjects. Eur J Clin Invest 1994;24 Suppl 3:31-5.

35. Viswanath V, Urooj A, Malleshi NG. Evaluation of antioxidant and antimicrobial properties of finger millet polyphenols (Eleusine coracana). Food Chem 2009;114:340-6.

Chapter-10

Nutraceutical and Health Properties of Psyllium

Introduction

Psyllium encompasses mucilaginous materials derived from the seeds and seed husks of various Plantago genus plants, including P. ovata, P. psyllium, and P. indica. This substance is cultivated in specific sub-tropical regions across Asia, North Africa, and parts of Europe's Mediterranean regions. The composition of psyllium comprises a densely substituted acidic arabinoxylan. Its xylan backbone exhibits both (β 1 $\to$ 4) and (β 1 $\to$ 3) linkages, accompanied by single xylopyranosyl branches at C-2 and trisaccharide side chains at C-3 positions. The identified trisaccharide side chains consist of L-Araf-α-(1 $\to$ 3)-D-Xylp-β-(1 $\to$ 3)-L-Araf, as confirmed through NMR and methylation studies. Other monosaccharides detected in psyllium include D-galactose, D-galacturonic acid, D-rhamnose, 4-O-methyl-D-glucuronic acid, and 2-O-(2-D-galactopyranosyluronic acid)-L-rhamnose.

Psyllium serves as a health component in food, dietary supplements, cosmetics, and pharmaceutical products, including lotions and drug delivery systems. It has been employed in managing conditions like constipation, diarrhea, and weight control while potentially reducing the risk of cardiovascular diseases, irritable bowel syndrome, inflammation, and colon cancer. Additionally, psyllium finds application as a functional ingredient in various consumer products, functioning as a deflocculant in paper and textile manufacturing and a binder in meat products. Moreover, derivatives of psyllium polysaccharides have been studied for their role as oral delivery systems for bioactive components. This overview delves into the health attributes of psyllium, its potential biological mechanisms, the impact of structural modifications on its functions, and the potential adverse effects associated with psyllium intake.

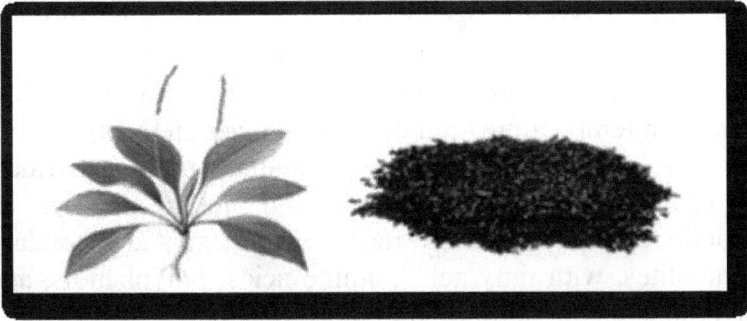

Figure 1: The Plantago genus plant (left), and traditional Chinese herb Che Qian Zi/psyllium (right).

Chemical constituents

Psyllium refers to the seeds of an annual herb belonging to the Plantago genus, which includes numerous species like Plantago ovata Forssk., Plantago asiatica L., Plantago major L., and Plantago depressa Willd. This genus is widely distributed across temperate and high-elevation tropical regions. Once harvested, the husk, a white membranous covering constituting approximately 30% of the dried seed's weight, is separated from the seed through milling.

Comprising soluble (predominantly arabinoxylans) and insoluble polysaccharides (hemicellulose, cellulose, and lignin), psyllium and its husk also contain tannins, phenols, and flavonoids. The husk, a blend of neutral and acid polysaccharides containing galacturonic acid, boasts a soluble/insoluble fiber ratio of 70/30. The notable health benefits and food applications of psyllium and its husk largely stem from their high arabinoxylan content, particularly more concentrated in the husk. Psyllium polysaccharides, a significant bioactive ingredient extracted from the seeds, consist of xylose, arabinose, galactose, rhamnose, glucose, and mannose in varying molar ratios. These polysaccharides have shown diverse health-promoting effects such as antioxidant, antitumor, immunomodulatory, anti-proliferative, hypoglycemic, hypotensive, and antiviral activities.

It's important to note that factors like raw materials, extraction temperature, and duration impact the composition, structure, and functionality of psyllium polysaccharides. Moreover, both psyllium seeds and husks are rich in bioactive compounds and a range of primary and secondary metabolites, with fatty acids, amino acids, polyphenols, and flavonoids being among the most abundant. Specifically, polyphenols and flavonoids with antioxidant properties hold potential for addressing diseases triggered by excessive reactive oxygen species (ROS).

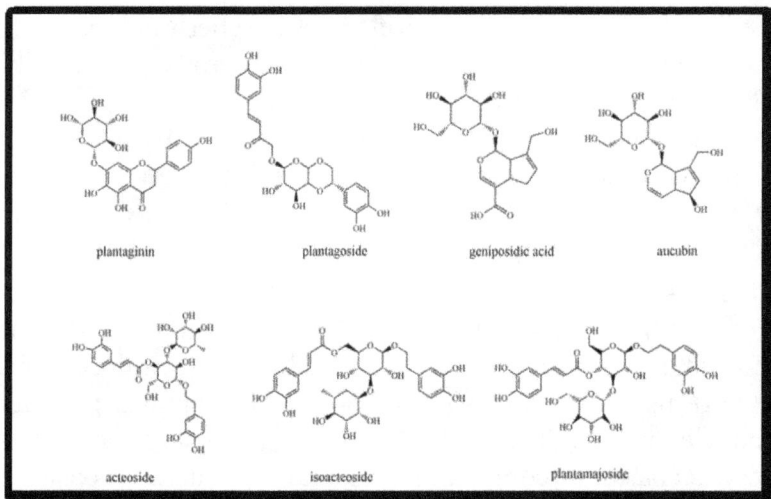

Figure 2: Chemical structures of the representative components of psyllium

Psyllium applications in food systems

The growing awareness of a healthy diet has led to an increasing demand for functional food, which has induced the food industry to search for new functional products with health benefits. Meanwhile, the sensory properties, such as color, flavor, texture, and overall acceptability, will affect consumers' acceptance. According to previous studies, some researchers have added psyllium husk into food products (such as ice cream, biscuits, gluten-free bread, noodles, pizza, pasta, and cakes), and reported health benefits such as cholesterol control, glycemic control, and satiety, among others . In addition, the addition of psyllium has been shown to obtain a softer crumb in high-fiber wheat bread and improve dough mechanical properties and gluten-free bread shelf-life. However, the incorporation of psyllium husk in different foods is limited, as high levels of fiber may cause disagreeable changes in the texture and color of foods. Particularly in baked products, it was observed that cookies with psyllium husk were darker than those without it. Thus, further research may focus on minimizing the undesired effects of a great incorporation of psyllium husk in food to improve its quality and consumer acceptability.

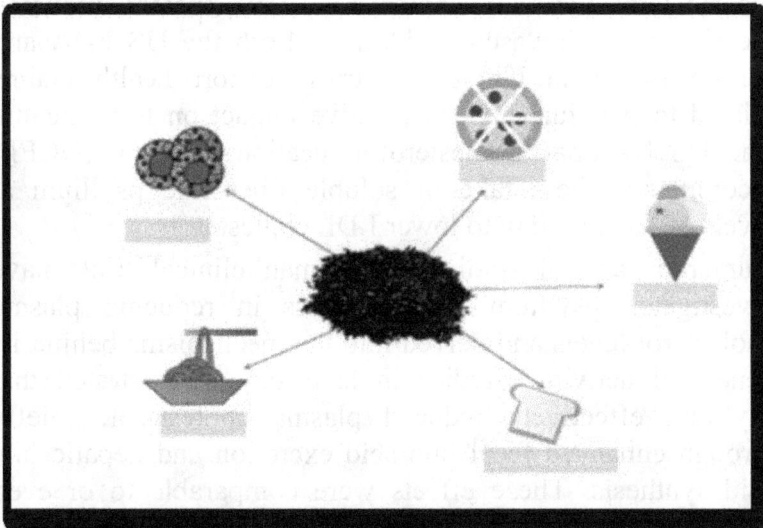

Figure 3: Psyllium applications in food systems.

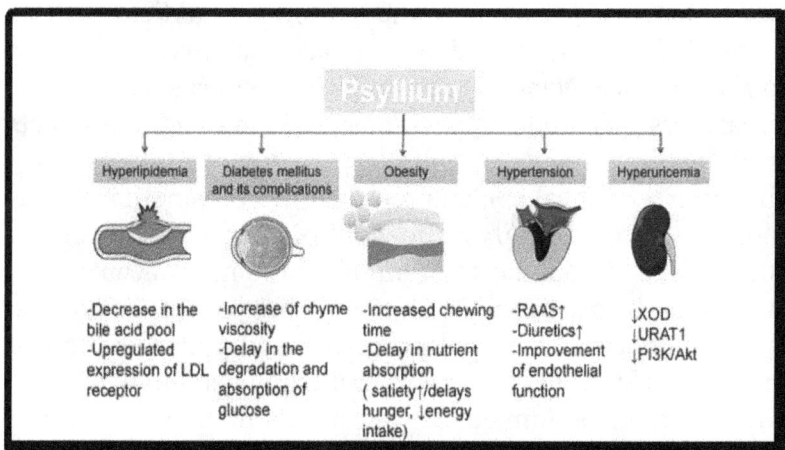

Figure 4: Health beneficial effects of psyllium

An overview of the major beneficial effects of psyllium

Hypolipidemic effect

Dietary fibers, particularly soluble fibers from psyllium seed husks, have gained recognition for their potential to reduce plasma total and LDL cholesterol levels, thereby reducing the risk of cardiovascular diseases. Both the US FDA and certain European Union countries support health claims related to psyllium and its positive impact on heart health. The US National Cholesterol Education Program (NCEP) recommends the intake of soluble fiber like psyllium at levels of 10–25 g/day to lower LDL cholesterol.

Numerous animal studies and human clinical trials have investigated psyllium's effectiveness in reducing plasma cholesterol levels and delved into the mechanisms behind its beneficial activity. Studies in hamsters demonstrated that psyllium effectively reduced plasma cholesterol, chiefly through enhanced fecal bile acid excretion and hepatic bile acid synthesis. These effects were comparable to or even more pronounced than those of other dietary fibers like pectin and guar gum. Modified psyllium preparations also exhibited heightened hypocholesterolemic effects in animal models.

Consistent with animal studies, research on rats, mice, guinea pigs, and monkeys echoed psyllium's ability to reduce cholesterol concentrations, emphasizing increased fecal bile acid excretion and alterations in various enzyme activities associated with cholesterol metabolism.

Human studies further affirmed psyllium's cholesterol-lowering effects. These trials showcased significant reductions in total plasma cholesterol and LDL cholesterol levels in hypercholesterolemic subjects consuming psyllium. Similar outcomes were observed in studies comparing psyllium with other dietary fibers, with psyllium proving particularly effective in improving lipid profiles. Notably, psyllium-enriched diets also exhibited positive effects in patients with non-insulin dependent diabetes mellitus and hyperlipidemia, as well as in individuals with cardiovascular disease.

The mechanisms behind psyllium's cholesterol-lowering effects involve multiple pathways, including increased bile acid binding, disruption of micelle formation in the intestine, modulation of lipid metabolism-related genes, and potential influences on hormonal status, insulin resistance, and intestinal motility. These mechanisms may work collectively or independently to achieve the observed cholesterol-lowering benefits.

In summary, psyllium has demonstrated promising potential in reducing total and LDL cholesterol levels, as well as total serum triglycerides, while increasing HDL cholesterol. While some mechanisms like bile acid binding and micelle disruption are suggested, ongoing research aims to uncover the precise mechanisms driving psyllium's beneficial effects on cholesterol.

Hypoglycaemic effect

Psyllium has demonstrated efficacy in improving postprandial glycemic index and insulin sensitivity in various studies. For instance, recent research indicated that the hot-water extractable components of Plantago ovata at 0.5 g/kg body weight/day notably suppressed the increase in blood glucose levels triggered by the oral intake of glucose or sucrose in rats. Interestingly, this effect was observed without affecting fasting blood glucose levels and insulin status. Psyllium was found to reduce sucrose absorption in the gastrointestinal tract, limit intestinal glucose absorption during perfusion, and enhance gastrointestinal motility. However, it did not impact disaccharidase activity, suggesting its role in reducing hyperglycemia might involve suppressing intestinal glucose absorption.

In earlier studies, psyllium exhibited the ability to enhance blood glucose disposal and improve insulin sensitivity by significantly increasing skeletal muscle plasma membrane GLUT-4 protein expression in stroke-prone spontaneously hypertensive rats. GLUT-4 protein plays a crucial role in glucose transportation into skeletal muscle, and psyllium appeared to facilitate glucose uptake by increasing the presence of this transporter without activating phospha-tidylinositol 3-kinase, a usual signaling pathway for GLUT-4 translocation.

Numerous reports highlight psyllium's potential to decrease postprandial glucose and insulin concentrations in individuals with diabetes, hypercholesterolemia, hyper-tension, and obesity. An early study involving non-insulin-dependent diabetic patients demonstrated that psyllium intake before meals reduced postprandial glucose elevation significantly at breakfast and dinner, as well as after lunch, compared to a placebo. This effect was linked to psyllium's capacity to form a strong gel, which affected fluid viscosity in the gastrointestinal system. Recent human studies further supported these findings, illustrating that dietary psyllium intake reduced postprandial serum glucose and insulin concentrations in hypercholesterolemic men and type 2 diabetic individuals.

Studies using 5.1 g of psyllium per day for two weeks revealed notable reductions in post-lunch postprandial glucose concentrations in men with type 2 diabetes. Longer treatment durations with psyllium, such as an eight-week regimen of 5.1 g psyllium twice daily, demonstrated significant reductions in fasting plasma glucose and glycosylated hemoglobin (HbA1c) levels in type 2 diabetic patients. More recent investigations confirmed that a two-month treatment with psyllium led to decreased fasting plasma glucose, HbA1c levels, triglycerides, and blood pressure in individuals with type 2 diabetes.

However, conflicting results exist regarding the residual effects of psyllium after the second meal in type 2 diabetic patients. Overall, these studies indicate that incorporating psyllium into a regular diet is safe and unlikely to adversely affect the bioavailability of dietary minerals and vitamins.

Effects in gastrointestinal system

Psyllium is widely acknowledged for its remarkable laxative properties. In a study conducted in 1998 involving 170 subjects, psyllium was found to be more effective than docusate sodium as a stool softener and laxative for the treatment of chronic idiopathic constipation. This study demonstrated that psyllium intake at a dose of 5.1 g twice daily over two weeks led to increased stool water content, total stool output, and frequency of bowel movements. These beneficial effects might be attributed to psyllium's capacity to hold and absorb water.

Further investigations confirmed the laxative effects of psyllium. An examination using human subjects revealed that an unfermented gel-forming component of psyllium in the colon contributed to the formation of bulkier and more moist stools, thereby facilitating laxation. Psyllium was also noted to augment the excretion of short-chain fatty acids in stools without significantly altering the mass of fecal bacteria. Changes in the pH of the colon could be another contributing factor to psyllium's laxative effects.

Interestingly, psyllium exhibits paradoxical properties, being capable of alleviating both constipation and diarrhea. Studies have shown that psyllium husk delays gastric emptying and reduces the speed of colon transit by increasing meal viscosity and slowing down the formation of gaseous products resulting from colon fermentation.

Moreover, research studies exploring the potential use of psyllium for irritable bowel syndrome (IBS), a common gastrointestinal disorder characterized by recurrent abdominal pain or discomfort and changes in bowel habits, have indicated promising results. Previous findings suggest that psyllium may offer a viable treatment option for individuals with IBS.

Cancer prevention

Research, particularly by Yu and colleagues in 2009, has reviewed the potential role of psyllium in cancer prevention, notably colon and breast cancers. In a study by Morita et al. in 1999, psyllium, when incorporated at a level of 15 g/kg in the diet, redirected high-amylose corn starch fermentation toward the distal colon in rats. This dietary change resulted in increased fecal butyrate content. Butyrate, a crucial short-chain fatty acid, holds promise in preventing colon cancer by potentially suppressing cancer cell proliferation, enhancing differentiation marker expression, and causing neoplastic cell reversion to a nonneoplastic state.

Additionally, psyllium might influence colonic sphingomyelin metabolism and apoptosis, impacting colon tumorigenesis and inflammation in mice. Studies with psyllium extract and pure β-sitosterol from psyllium extract revealed their ability to restore gap junctional intercellular communication in rat liver cells transfected with Ha-ras. Upregulation of this communication is linked to several anticarcinogenic compounds.

However, conflicting evidence exists regarding the preventive effects of psyllium on colon cancer. Ma et al. scrutinized available data and suggested that psyllium and other soluble fibers, such as pectin, might not significantly reduce the risk of colon cancer.

In the context of breast cancer prevention, a study in F344 rats evaluated different combinations of psyllium and wheat bran in various ratios in the diet. The 4%:4% (wheat bran/psyllium) diet demonstrated the lowest mammary tumorigenesis after a 19-week treatment period. Notably, higher psyllium intake correlated with reduced fecal estrogen excretion. However, differences in circulating and urinary estrogen levels among rats on various diets were not detected. Psyllium intake also suppressed bacterial β-D glucuronidase activity, yet the precise relationship between this activity and mammary tumor development remains unclear. Other phytochemicals like phytates, isoflavonoids, and proteinase inhibitors might contribute to the overall anticancer effects. Further research is needed to explore whether a combination of insoluble and soluble fiber could offer a more effective strategy for reducing the risk of mammary cancer.

Anti-inflammation effect

A study aimed to explore the impact of psyllium on inflammatory markers, specifically C-reactive protein (CRP), a marker linked to dietary fiber intake. CRP serves as an independent predictor for cardiovascular disease and is associated with various health issues like diabetes and hypertension. Interestingly, in this study conducted on overweight or obese adults, no significant differences in inflammatory markers, including CRP, fibrinogen, and IL-6, were observed between the group receiving psyllium treatment and the control group.

This finding aligns with a recent study by North et al. in 2009, which also concluded that while increased fiber intake reduced CRP levels, supplementation specifically with psyllium did not exhibit the same effect. However, further research is essential to delve into the effect of psyllium on CRP specifically in healthy human subjects.

Obesity

Psyllium, recognized as an effective means to address obesity, operates by regulating appetite, reducing energy intake, and consequently aiding weight loss in various clinical and epidemiological studies. With the global prevalence of obesity anticipated to escalate, the association between obesity and cardiovascular diseases (CVDs) remains a growing concern, drawing attention to psyllium's potential benefits.

Studies reveal that psyllium's ability to form a gel in the small intestine delays digestion and absorption, fostering a feeling of fullness and diminishing hunger, thereby curbing energy intake and promoting weight reduction. Clinical trials assessing psyllium's impact on satiety consistently demonstrate reductions in hunger and an increase in fullness between meals compared to placebos. Psyllium's effectiveness in moderating hunger feelings, limiting food intake, and mitigating postprandial fluctuations in glucose and insulin levels has been observed.

Moreover, in clinical investigations, psyllium supplementation exhibited promising outcomes in overweight and obese individuals, resulting in reductions in body weight, BMI, and waist circumference, along with improvements in non-alcoholic fatty liver disease (NAFLD) markers. Notably, studies in patients with type 2 diabetes and chronic constipation reported significant weight reduction with psyllium supplementation compared to placebos.

However, despite its potential in modulating inflammatory markers linked to obesity-related cardiovascular risks, findings regarding psyllium's impact on certain inflammatory markers like C-reactive protein (CRP) remain inconclusive. While some studies indicate a reduction in inflammatory markers, others demonstrate no significant effect, suggesting the need for further investigation. Psyllium's potential in influencing pro-inflammatory and anti-inflammatory adipokines, hence addressing chronic inflammation associated with obesity-driven CVDs, has been highlighted in various studies, showcasing its therapeutic promise.

In summary, psyllium's multifaceted benefits include appetite suppression, energy intake regulation, weight reduction, and a potential role in modulating inflammatory markers and adipokines to combat obesity-related chronic inflammation linked to cardiovascular diseases.

Top of Form

Potential in controlled delivery of bioactives

The investigation into cross-linked polysaccharide derivatives from Plantago psyllium mucilage and Plantago ovate husks has shown promise in the oral delivery of bioactive compounds. These derivatives, being gel-forming and edible polysaccharides, present fewer safety concerns, making them appealing for consumption. Different methods, such as chemical polymerization agents or radiation-initiated polymerization, have been utilized to create cross-link networks in these polysaccharides.

Agents like acrylic acid derivatives such as methacrylamide (MAAm) and N,N'-methylenebisacrylamide (MBAAm) have been instrumental in forming novel cross-linked psyllium derivatives. These cross-linked polymers have exhibited potential as a targeted delivery system for various bioactive compounds, including drugs like rifampicin and 5-

fluoruracil, specifically to the colon. The release of these drugs from the hydrogel systems followed a non-Fickian diffusion model, offering controlled and sustained delivery. Chemical inducers like ammonium persulphate (APS) have also played a role in polymerization processes, forming hydrogels that effectively deliver compounds such as tetracycline hydrochloric acid to the colon. Moreover, psyllium derivatives treated with polycarboxylic acids have demonstrated the capability to modulate the release of drugs like diltiazem-HCl in tablet formulations.

While these findings are promising, further research directly comparing psyllium-based oral hydrogels with established colon-targeted delivery systems using a broader range of bioactives, including drugs with diverse chemical and physical properties, is necessary to validate and expand these applications.

Possible adverse effects

Though generally considered safe for consumption, psyllium intake has been associated with various adverse effects. These include reduced caloric availability, suppressed appetite, bloating, flatulence, potential abdominal pain, anaphylactic symptoms, and altered nutrient and drug absorption. Research has shown that psyllium intake might decrease the absorption of substances like riboflavin and inhibit iron absorption, while its effects on calcium absorption have varied across studies. Animal studies indicated reduced calcium bioavailability and negative impacts on bone composition due to psyllium intake, but human studies at therapeutic levels suggested minimal effects on calcium availability when co-ingested. Psyllium's viscosity and fermentability play a role in its impact on mineral absorption; lower viscosity and fermentability may result in less inhibition of calcium, magnesium, and zinc absorption.

Allergic reactions to psyllium seeds were observed among healthcare workers with daily exposure, indicating sensitization and clinical allergy rates. Psyllium ingestion has been linked to increased gas production, slower intestinal gas transit, and associated symptoms like abdominal distension, pain, flatulence, and bloating. Moreover, it has been noted to suppress caloric intake over a period and has demonstrated cholesterol-lowering, glucose-lowering, and laxative effects. While showing potential for treating conditions like IBS, its potential cancer prevention and anti-inflammatory effects require further confirmation. Researchers are exploring modified psyllium preparations with altered properties for potential use in managing hypercholesterolemia while reducing viscosity and gel-forming characteristics.

Conclusions

Due to its considerable medicinal and economic significance, psyllium, particularly its husk, has garnered substantial attention from researchers. The husks are packed with dietary fiber known for its high viscosity, solubility in water, and superior gel-forming abilities, offering a long history of health benefits. These benefits encompass the prevention and management of various common diseases such as hyperlipidemia, diabetes, obesity, cardiovascular issues, constipation, irritable bowel syndrome, diarrhea, and potentially cancer, many of which are linked to cardiometabolic disorders (CMDs).

Both observational and experimental studies highlight that the positive effects and diverse applications of psyllium largely stem from its viscosity. When psyllium interacts with water, it creates a viscous gel that binds to bile acids in the gut, aiding in their elimination through stools. This process supports the conversion of cholesterol into bile acids, ultimately lowering blood cholesterol levels. The gel's viscosity slows down interactions between digestive enzymes and nutrients in the gastrointestinal system, delaying the breakdown and absorption of glucose and other nutrients, thereby assisting in blood sugar management. This delayed digestion and absorption contribute to prolonged satiety, reducing energy intake and aiding weight loss in overweight or obese individuals. Importantly, the water-holding capacity and gel-forming properties of psyllium fiber rely on its viscosity.

Prior research has also indicated that psyllium and its extracts may directly or indirectly lower blood pressure and improve cardiac hypertrophy induced by prolonged hypertension. Hyperuricemia, increasingly recognized as a significant risk factor alongside hypertension, hyperlipidemia, and hyperglycemia, poses cardiovascular risks often associated with these conditions. Studies have shown the potential of psyllium and its extracts in treating hyperuricemia, suggesting their therapeutic role. However, further exploration is needed to fully understand the mechanisms underlying psyllium's ability to lower uric acid levels, potentially paving the way for more effective pharmaceutical strategies for CMD treatment using psyllium.

References
1. Anderson, J.W., Jones , A.E., and Riddellmason, S. (1994) 10 different dietary-fibers have significantly different effects on serum and liver lipids of cholesterol-fed rats . Journal of Nutrition , 124 : 78 – 83 .
2. Anderson, J., Allgood , L.D. , Turner , J. , Oeltgen , P.R., and Daggy , B.P. (1999) Effects of psyllium on glucose and serum lipid responses in men with type 2 diabetes and hypercholesterolemia. American Journal of Clinical Nutrition , 70 : 466 – 473 .

3. Agrawal , A.R., Tandon, M., and Sharma, P.L. (2007) Effect of combining viscous fibre with lovastatin on serum lipids in normal human subjects . International Journal of Clinical Practice , 61 : 1812 – 1818
4. Bijkerk , C.J., de Wit, N.J., Muris , J.W.M. , Whorwell , P.J., Knottnerus , J.A. , and Hoes , A.W. (2009) Soluble or insoluble fibre in irritable bowel syndrome in primary care? Randomised placebo controlled trial . British Medical Journal , 339 : b3956 .
5. Bliss, D.Z., Jung , H.J. , Savik , K. , Lowry , A. , LeMoine, M., Jensen, L., Werner, C., and Schaffer, K. (2001) Supplementation with dietary fiber improves fecal incontinence. Nursing Research, 50 : 203–213. Chan, M.Y. and Heng, C.K. (2008) Sequential effects of a high-fiber diet with psyllium husks on the expression levels of hepatic genes and plasma lipids . Nutrition , 24 : 57 – 66 .
6. Chen , W.J.L., Anderson, J.W., and Jennings, D. (1984) Propionate May Mediate the Hypocholesterolemic Effects of Certain Soluble Plant Fibers in Cholesterol-Fed Rats . Proceedings of the Society for Experimental Biology and Medicine , 175 : 215 – 218 .
7. Cheng, Y.J., Ohlsson, L., and Duan, R.D. (2004) Psyllium and fat in diets differentially affect the activities and expressions of colonic sphingomyelinases and caspase in mice . British Journal of Nutrition , 91 : 715 – 723 .
8. Cheng, Z., Blackford, J., Wang, Q., and Yu L. (2009) Acid treatment to improve psyllium functionality . Journal of Functional Foods , 1 : 44 – 49 .
9. Cicero, A.F.G., Derosa, G., Manca, M., Bove, M., Borghi, C., and Gaddi, A.V. (2007) Different effect of psyllium and guar dietary supplementation on blood pressure control in hypertensive overweight patients: A six-month, randomized clinical trial. Clinical and Experimental Hypertension , 29 : 383 – 394 .
10. Cohen, L.A., Zhao, Z.L., Zang, E.A., Wynn, T.T., Simi, B., and Rivenson, A. (1996) Wheat bran and psyllium

diets: Effects on N-methylnitrosourea-induced mammary tumorigenesis in F344 rats. Journal of the National Cancer Institute , 88 : 899 – 907 .

11. Everson, G.T., Daggy, B.P., McKinley, C., and Story, J.A. (1992) Effects of psyllium hydrophilic mucilloid on LDL-cholesterol and bile acid synthesis in hypercholesterolemic men . Journal of Lipid Research , 33 : 1183 – 1192 .

12. Fernandez, R. and Phillips, S.F. (1982a) Components of Fiber Bind Iron Invitro. American Journal of Clinical Nutrition , 35 : 100 – 106 .

13. Fernandez, R. and Phillips, S.F. (1982b) Components of Fiber Impair Iron-Absorption in the Dog. American Journal of Clinical Nutrition , 35 : 107 – 112 .

14. Fly, A.D., CzarneckiMaulden, G.L., Fahey, G.C., and Titgemeyer, E.C. (1996) Hemicellulose does not affect iron bioavailability in chicks . Journal of Nutrition , 126 : 308 – 316 .

15. Ganji, V. and Kuo, J. (2008) Serum lipid responses to psyllium fiber: differences between pre- and postmenopausal, hypercholesterolemic women . Nutrition Journal , 7 : 22 .

16. Gohel , M.C. , Amin , A.F. , Chhabaria , M.T. , Panchal , M.K. , and Lalwani , A.N. (2000) Modulation of drug release rate of diltiazem-HCl from hydrogel matrices of succinic acid-treated ispaghula husk . Pharmaceutical Development and Technology , 5 : 375 – 381 .

17. Gohel, M.C., Patel, M.M., and Amin, A.F. (2003) Development of modified release diltiazem HCl tablets using composite index to identify optimal formulation . Drug Development and Industrial Pharmacy , 29 : 565 – 574 .

18. Gupta, R.R., Agrawal, C.G., Singh, G.P., and Ghatak , A. (1994) Lipid-lowering efficacy of psyllium hydrophilic mucilloid in non insulin dependent diabetes mellitus with

hyperlipidaemia. India Journal of Medicine Research , 100 : 237 – 241 .
19. Heaney, R.P. and Weaver, C.M. (1995) Effect of psyllium on absorption of co-ingested calcium . Journal of the American Geriatrics Society , 43 : 261 – 263 .
20. Jalihal, A. and Kurian, G. (1990) Ispaghula therapy in irritable-bowel-syndrome – improvement in overall well-being is related to reduction in bowel dissatisfaction . Journal of Gastro enterology and Hepatology , 5 : 507 – 513 .
21. Jenkins, D.J.A., Kendall, C.W.C., Vuksan, V., Vidgen, E., Parker, T., Faulkner, D., Mehling, C.C., Garsetti, M , Testolin, G., Cunnane, S.C., Ryan, M.A., and Corey, P.N. (2002) Soluble fiber intake at a dose approved by the US Food and Drug Administration for a claim of health benefits: serum lipid
22. Sprecher, D.L., Harris, B.V., Goldberg , A.C., Anderson, E.C., Bayuk , L.M. , Russell, B.S., Crone, D.S., Quinn, C. , Bateman, J., Kuzmak, B.R., and Allgood, L.D. (1993) Efficacy of psyllium in reducing serum cholesterol levels in hypercholesterolemic patients on high- or low-fat diets . Annals of Internal Medicine , 119 (1): 545 – 554 .
23. Stoy, D.B., LaRosa, J.C., Brewer, B.K., Mackey, M., and Meusing, R.A. (1993) Cholesterol-lowering effects of ready-to-eat cereal containing psyllium. Journal of the American Dietetic Association , 93 : 910 – 912 .
24. Terpstra, A.H.M., Lapre, J.A., de Vries, H.T., and Beynen, A.C. (2000) Hypocholesterolemic effect of dietary psyllium in female rats . Annals of Nutrition and Metabolism , 44 : 223 – 238 .
25. Vega-Lopez , S., Vidal-Quintanar, R.L., and Fernandez, M.L. (2001) Sex and hormonal status influence plasma lipid responses to psyllium. American Journal of Clinical Nutrition , 74 : 435 – 441 .

26. Vega-Lopez, S., Conde-Knape, K., Vidal-Quintanar, R.L., Shachter, N.S., and Fernandez, M.L. (2002) Sex and hormonal status influence the effects of psyllium on lipoprotein remodeling and composition . Metabolism-Clinical and Experimental , 51 : 500 – 507 .
27. Vega-Lopez, S., Freake, H.C., and Fernandez, M.L. (2003) Sex and hormonal status modulate the effects of psyllium on plasma lipids and monocyte gene expression in humans. Journal of Nutrition , 133 : 67 – 70 .
28. Wär, J., Marcos, A., Bueno, G., and Moreno, L.A. (2009) Functional benefits of psyllium fiber supplementation . Current Topics in Nutraceutical Research , 7 : 55 – 63 .
29. Wei, Z.H., Wang, H., Chen, X.Y., Wang, B.S., Rong, Z.X., Wang, B.S., Su, B.H., and Chen, H.Z. (2009) Time- and dose-dependent effect of psyllium on serum lipids in mild-to-moderate hypercholesterolemia: a meta-analysis of controlled clinical trials . European Journal of Clinical Nutrition , 63 : 821 – 827 .
30. Yu, L.L., Lutterodt, H., and Cheng, Z. (2009) Beneficial health properties of psyllium and approaches to improve its functionalities. Advances in Food and Nutrition Research , 55 : 193 – 220

Chapter-11

Nutraceutical and Health Properties of Common Beans (Phaseolus Vulgaris)

Introduction

The common bean, scientifically known as Phaseolus vulgaris L., holds a significant historical legacy as one of the earliest cultivated crops globally. This herbaceous annual legume boasts substantial genetic diversity, with various races originating from Middle America and Andean South America. Over time, it has transformed from a wild-growing vine into a staple dietary legume, now cultivated far beyond its original regions (Schoonhoven and Voysest, 1991).

Similar to other legumes, the common bean engages in a symbiotic relationship, allowing it to obtain nitrogen. This trait enables various varieties of this plant to act as nitrogen-fixing organisms, forming nodules with diverse rhizobial strains. Consequently, it serves as a crucial protein source, particularly for populations in Latin America (Vásquez-Arroyo et al., 1998).

Presently, both dry and green beans are cultivated worldwide, with a broad spectrum of top production sites across different geographical regions. In 2008 alone, global production tallied around 18 million metric tons, solidifying the common bean's status as the most economically significant variety within the Phaseolus genus. Among the pulse food legumes, it stands out as the most extensive and widely consumed.Varieties within P. vulgaris encompass black beans, white beans, pinto beans, and kidney beans (see Figure 1), playing pivotal roles as primary sources of dietary protein in numerous developing nations.

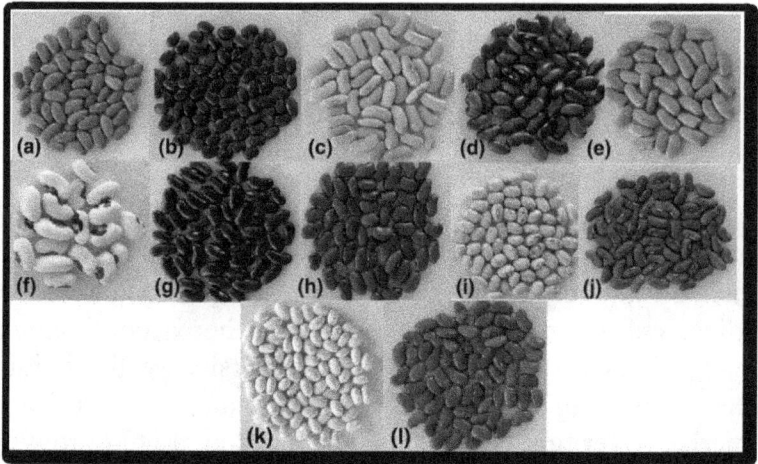

Figure 1 : Different types of common beans with different seat coat colour

Health beneficial effects of Phaseolus vulgaris

The consumption of common bean extract has shown promise in alleviating symptoms associated with chronic conditions, notably diabetes and obesity. Additionally, the dietary common bean has exhibited hypocholesterolemic properties, potentially reducing the risk of coronary heart disease. Studies have also indicated that P. vulgaris may have anticarcinogenic effects in animal models.

These health benefits linked to common bean consumption are likely due to its rich array of functional components. The bean contains various phytochemicals, including phenolic compounds, dietary fiber, and alpha-amylase inhibitors. Phenolic compounds, for instance, are recognized for their anti-carcinogenic and antioxidant properties, as shown in Figure 2. Antioxidants play a crucial role as potent scavengers of free radicals and reactive oxygen species, effectively impeding oxidative processes that contribute to chronic diseases. Therefore, the common bean serves as a natural source of antioxidants, initiating these positive health effects.

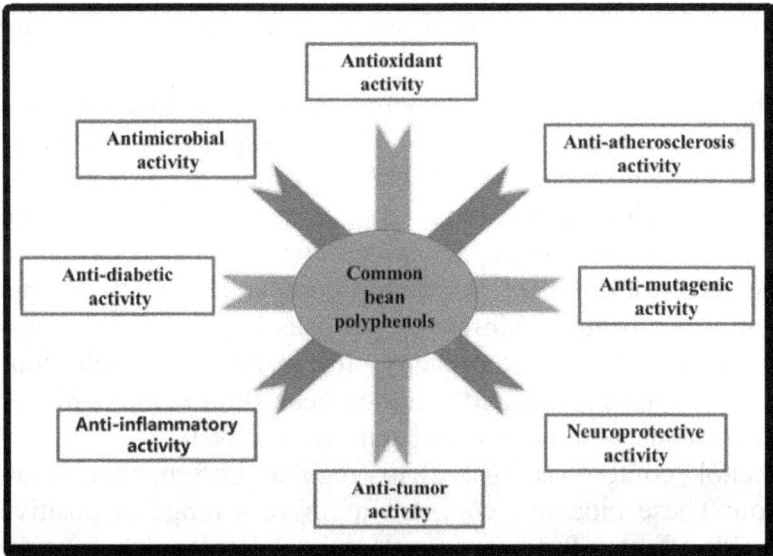

Figure 2 : Health benefits of common bean polyphenols

Natural antioxidants in the common bean

Numerous studies have highlighted the abundant presence of antioxidants in various common bean varieties, particularly concentrated in their seed coats. The total phenolic content in hull, whole, and dehulled beans has been measured, ranging from 0.6 to 78.2 mg of catechin equivalents per gram of sample. Notably, bean hulls exhibit substantially higher phenolic content and antioxidant activity compared to whole beans. For example, manually separated hulls display a 37-fold greater phenolic content than whole bean flour and dehulled beans.

Phenolic compounds, notably quercetin, kaempferol, flavonols, daidzein, anthocyanins, and tannins, constitute the majority of antioxidants in the common bean. Quercetin and kaempferol content in whole beans range from 6.9–23.5 and 13.8–204 µg/g bean, respectively. Additionally, four phenolic acids—p-hydroxybenzoic acid, vanillic acid, p-coumaric acid, and ferulic acid—are detected in varying quantities, with ferulic acid predominating at 17 to 36 µg/g bean.

The antioxidant and polyphenol content fluctuates among different common bean genotypes, corresponding to varying levels of antioxidant activity. Mutants induced by NaN3, for instance, show significantly higher accumulations of total phenols, anthocyanins, and preanthocyanidins, resulting in elevated antioxidant capacity compared to traditional common beans. Moreover, processing methods also influence antioxidant capacity; for instance, tempeh flour obtained from fermented common bean flour exhibits higher antioxidant and antiradical activity, as well as increased phenol content compared to regular unfermented bean flour.These bioactive components drive a range of positive health effects. Tannins, prevalent in red-colored beans, are polyphenolic compounds with diverse bioactivities including anti-inflammatory, antiproliferative, and antimicrobial functions. They serve as potent antioxidants with free radical-scavenging abilities, metal-chelating activity, and the capacity to inhibit lipid peroxidation and prooxidative enzymes.

Anthocyanins, another group of antioxidants present in beans, act not only as pigments but also possess antioxidant properties, contributing to secondary health benefits such as anticarcinogenic and anti-inflammatory functions. They also play a beneficial role in managing diabetes and obesity, as well as in preventing cardiovascular disease.Finally, flavonols found in beans exhibit antioxidant effects and offer protective benefits for various health conditions.

Dietary fiber in the common bean

The dry common bean contains a rich blend of soluble and insoluble fiber, both of which are associated with various health benefits, particularly concerning cardiovascular health and digestive disorders. Interestingly, the positive effects of fiber on health appear to be influenced by its interaction with phytochemicals, a phenomenon likely evident in Phaseolus vulgaris. Studies assessing nutrient content in beans have consistently revealed significant levels of dietary fiber across different types of common beans. The total dietary fiber content in processed beans ranges between 10.97 and 48.1% of the bean's total weight, underscoring their importance as a dietary fiber source.

Research emphasizes the critical role of adequate fiber intake in preventing and managing chronic diseases. Increased intake of dietary fiber, especially soluble fiber, has been linked to reduced risks of coronary heart disease. Studies from the NHANES I study cohort indicated that a higher intake of soluble fiber, around 10–15 g daily, can notably lower total cholesterol and LDL-cholesterol levels. Common beans, known for their soluble fiber content, contribute to these cholesterol-lowering effects.

Moreover, higher dietary fiber intake correlates with reduced blood pressure and enhanced postprandial satiety, potentially aiding in weight management. Literature reviews suggest that different types of dietary fiber significantly influence energy intake by increasing feelings of fullness, satiation, and compliance with reduced-calorie diets.

Viscous fiber, found in common beans, plays a role in blood glucose control by slowing gastric emptying, digestion, and glucose absorption. Studies have highlighted the beneficial effects of fiber in managing both type 1 and type 2 diabetes. Evidence indicates that consuming 50 g of dietary fiber daily for six months resulted in improved glycemic control in type 1 diabetic patients. Similarly, high fiber intake has been associated with better blood sugar control and reduced insulin demand in type 2 diabetics.

Furthermore, dietary fiber consumption has been proposed to aid in preventing certain cancers. Prospective cohort studies have established a negative correlation between fiber intake and the development of colorectal cancer. Similarly, long-term studies have shown a link between higher fiber intake and a reduced risk of developing breast cancer in post-menopausal women. Considering these effects, legumes, including the common bean, are increasingly recognized as functional foods due to their cholesterol-lowering attributes, largely attributed to their high fiber content.

Anti-hyperglycemic effect

The hypoglycemic properties of the common bean have been acknowledged for quite some time, with bean pods historically utilized as traditional remedies for diabetes mellitus. While various animal studies have been conducted, human studies testing either a pure extract of the bean or the whole bean itself against diabetes indicators, particularly hyperglycemia, are limited.In early studies, administering a common bean complex to diabetic rabbit models led to a significant reduction in blood sugar levels. Similarly, gastric administration of Phaseolus vulgaris preparations in healthy rabbits resulted in decreased hyperglycemic peaks, indicating an anti-hyperglycemic effect.

Studies administering aqueous common bean extracts to diabetic rats showcased remarkable reductions in blood glucose levels and improvements in other diabetes-related parameters and hepatic carbohydrate enzyme levels. This effect was even significant when compared to a sulfonylurea-class antihyperglycemic agent, indicating the potency of the bean extract. Recent animal studies continued this trend, demonstrating reductions in blood glucose levels with purified pancreatic alpha-amylase inhibitors extracted from white beans, even in healthy animal groups.

However, the hypoglycemic effect seems more pronounced in diabetic animals compared to healthy ones. Although promising, this evidence is limited, emphasizing the necessity for further investigation, particularly clinical studies, to firmly establish the relationship between common bean consumption and glycemic regulation. Only a few human studies have explored the hypoglycemic or carbohydrate absorption-reducing effects of common beans. In one study comparing cooked common beans to bread in healthy subjects on a carbohydrate-rich diet, the beans resulted in a significantly lower glycemic response.

Phaseolus vulgaris appears to exhibit its antihyperglycemic activity through an alpha-amylase inhibitor identified within kidney bean seeds. This inhibitor, particularly the major form Alpha-AI, demonstrates human pancreatic alpha-amylase inhibition activity. The white kidney bean extract containing this inhibitor might serve to prevent or ameliorate conditions related to both diabetes and obesity by reducing glycemia and calorie intake.Moreover, recent research has highlighted the common bean among botanical products associated with increased lipogenesis in differentiating adipocytes, resembling the activity of troglitazone, an anti-diabetic pharmaceutical agent. This in-vitro trial partially elucidates the anti-diabetic potential attributed to Phaseolus vulgaris.

Weight loss

Over the past decade, researchers have explored the potential of the common bean to aid in weight reduction. While numerous trials have employed herbal preparations incorporating Phaseolus vulgaris, only a handful of randomized, double-blinded, placebo-controlled studies have specifically focused on the common bean as the sole active ingredient.

In one such study involving 60 overweight participants, a daily dose of 450 mg of common bean extract, identified as an alpha-amylase inhibitor, was administered for 30 days before a carbohydrate-rich meal. The treatment group exhibited significant reductions in body weight, fat mass, and various anthropometric measurements compared to the placebo group. Within 30 days, those receiving the extract experienced average reductions of 6.45 lbs in body weight, 10.45% in body fat, and notable decreases in waist and hip circumferences, while the placebo group showed minimal changes.

Udani et al. conducted two studies three years apart, observing the impact of common bean extract on carbohydrate absorption and weight loss. In the first study involving 27 obese participants, individuals receiving 1500 mg of Phase 2 twice a day with meals showed a trend toward weight loss after eight weeks, although not statistically significant. However, there were no adverse effects observed at this dose. In the second study with 25 healthy subjects, those receiving 1000 mg of white bean extract twice daily experienced weight loss, though not statistically significant compared to the placebo group. Nevertheless, when analyzed based on total carbohydrate intake from the diet, there was a significant difference in weight loss between the bean extract group and the placebo group in the highest carbohydrate-consuming category.

These findings suggest that Phaseolus vulgaris extract might contribute to weight loss, particularly in individuals consuming higher carbohydrate diets. However, due to limited literature and some non-statistically significant weight loss data, further long-term clinical studies involving larger participant groups are necessary to firmly establish the efficacy of the common bean or its extracts in weight loss programs. Additionally, comparative studies evaluating the effects and safety profiles of common bean extract versus widely-used pharmaceutical weight loss products would offer valuable insights into their respective impacts on weight loss and adverse effects.

Cardiovascular disease prevention

Over the past three decades, studies have consistently highlighted Phaseolus vulgaris' protective role against cardiovascular disease, primarily through its hypolipidemic effects. In the previously mentioned study, rats exhibited significant reductions in various circulating blood lipids after consuming common beans for 45 days. This included noteworthy decreases in total cholesterol, very-low-density lipoprotein cholesterol, low-density lipoprotein cholesterol, serum triglycerides, free fatty acids, and phospholipids. Pari and Venkateswaran confirmed these findings, highlighting the hypolipidemic effects of common bean intake in these animals, which also helped prevent diabetes-related fatty acid alterations.

Earlier studies suggested that hypercholesterolemic rats fed whole beans might experience reduced cholesterol levels, albeit with a likelihood of retention in the enterohepatic circulation. Conversely, rats given beans without hulls showed higher cholesterol output. Additionally, research involving young male adults indicated that consuming baked beans was associated with reduced total blood cholesterol, possibly due to decreased fat intake while on a bean-rich diet.

Cancer prevention

Several animal studies have linked common bean consumption to potential cancer prevention. Hangen and Bennink observed that rats consuming common beans had a reduced incidence of lab-induced colon cancer, displaying significantly fewer tumor formations compared to control groups. Another study later suggested that ingestion of a polysaccharide extract from common beans correlated inversely with the development of the same cancer in rats. This effect was attributed to the production of short-chain fatty acids, particularly butyrate, in the colon.

Given Phaseolus vulgaris' richness in antioxidants and their recognized protective effects against cancer, it's plausible that common beans possess certain chemopreventive functions. However, conclusive, evidence-based information is essential and can only be obtained through comprehensive studies, particularly clinical investigations. Further research could establish a definitive relationship between common beans and cancer, identifying the specific components responsible for this potential link, considering the diverse array of functional compounds present in beans.

For example, haemagglutinins, a component of interest, have undergone in vitro studies showing promising results over the last decade. Recent research involving purified haemagglutinin from Japanese Hokkaido red beans demonstrated a potent anti-proliferative effect on human hepatoma cells. However, it's noteworthy that this compound isn't stable at temperatures exceeding 90°C.

Possible adverse effects

Various common bean varieties contain the lectin phytohaemagglutinin, a compound that, in excessive amounts, can be toxic, disrupting cell metabolism and leading to reversible poisoning. However, soaking and cooking beans at high temperatures effectively reduce or eliminate most of this compound, preventing its harmful effects. Interestingly, phytohaemagglutinin extracted from beans serves medical purposes as a mitogen, stimulating T-lymphocyte cell division. Additionally, as previously indicated, it may serve as a powerful inhibitor of cancer cell proliferation.

Conclusion

Phaseolus vulgaris, the common bean, is not merely a basic dietary component but also a functional food with potential implications for health and well-being. As previously mentioned, its inclusion in diets holds promise for managing diabetes, preventing cardiovascular disease, and potentially mitigating cancer risks. Offering dietary fiber and an array of antioxidants, common beans contribute to these functions while offering additional health benefits. Considering these advantages and the established nutritional value of common beans, promoting their abundant inclusion in diets appears beneficial.

However, the existing literature on this subject is notably limited, warranting further extensive studies, especially clinical investigations. These studies are crucial in establishing a robust relationship between common bean consumption and health outcomes, ultimately guiding dietary guidelines. Given the widespread availability, relatively low cost, and overall safety of common beans, governmental and academic institutions could readily invest in research involving this crop to unravel its potential health benefits and optimize dietary recommendations.

References

1. Akond, G.M., Khandaker, L., Berthold, J., Gates, L., Peters, K., Delong, H., and Hossain, K. (2011) Anthocyanin, total polyphenols and antioxidant activity of common bean . American Journal of Food Technology , 6 : 385 – 394 .
2. Anderson , J., Story, L., Sieling, B., Chen, W., Petro, M., and Story, J. (1984) Hypocholesterolemic effects of oat-bran or bean intake for hypercholesterolemic men. The American Journal of Clinical Nutrition , 40 : 1146 – 1155
3. Aparicio-Fernandez, X., Manzo-Bonilla, L., and Loarca-Pina, G.F. (2005) Comparison of antimutagenic activity of phenolic compounds in newly harvested and stored common beans Phaseolus vulgaris against aflatoxin B1 . Journal of Food Science , 70 : S73 – S78 .

4. Bazzano, L.A., He, J., Ogden, L.G., Loria, C., Vupputuri, S., Myers, L., and Whelton, P.K. (2001) Legume consumption and risk of coronary heart disease in US men and women: NHANES I Epidemiologic Follow-up Study. Archives of Internal Medicine, 161 : 2573 – 2578.
5. Bazzano, L.A., He, J., Ogden, L.G., Loria, C.M., and Whelton, P.K. (2003) Dietary fiber intake and reduced risk of coronary heart disease in US men and women – The National Health and Nutrition Examination Survey I Epidemiologic Follow-up Study. Archives of Internal Medicine, 163 : 1897 – 1904
6. Beninger, C.W., and Hosfield, G.L. (2003) Antioxidant activity of extracts, condensed tannin fractions, and pure flavonoids from Phaseolus vulgaris L. seed coat color genotypes. Journal of Agricultural and Food Chemistry, 51 : 7879 – 7883.
7. Blair, M., Torres, M., Giraldo, M., and Pedraza, F. (2009) Development and diversity of Andean-derived, gene-based microsatellites for common bean (Phaseolus vulgaris L.). BMC Plant Biology, 9 : 100
8. Celleno, L., Tolaini, M.V., D'Amore, A., Perricone, N.V., and Preuss, H.G. (2007) A dietary supplement containing standardized Phaseolus vulgaris extract influences body composition of overweight men and women. International Journal of Medical Sciences, 4 : 45 – 52.
9. Center for Food Safety and Applied Nutrition. (2009) The Bad Bug Book Foodborne Pathogenic Microorganisms and Natural Toxins Handbook. College Park, Md. : U.S. Food and Drug Administration.
10. Diaz, A.M., Caldas, G.V., and Blair, M.W. (2010) Concentrations of condensed tannins and anthocyanins in common bean seed coats. Food Research International, 43 : 595 – 601.
11. Díaz-Batalla, L., Widholm, J.M., Fahey, G.C., Castaño-Tostado, E., and Paredes-López, O. (2006) Chemical

components with health implications in wild and cultivated mexican common bean seeds (Phaseolus vulgaris L.) . Journal of Agricultural and Food Chemistry , 54 : 2045 – 2052 .

12. Feregrino-Perez, A.A., Berumen , L.C., Garcia-Alcocer, G., Guevara-Gonzalez, R.G., Ramos-Gomez , M. , Reynoso-Camacho, R., Acosta-Gallegos, J.A., and Loarca-Pina, G. (2008) Composition and chemopreventive effect of polysaccharides from common beans (Phaseolus vulgaris L.) on azoxymethane-induced colon cancer . Journal of Agricultural Food Chemistry , 56 : 8737 – 8744 .

13. Food and Agricultural Organization of the United Nations. (2009) FAOSTAT . Giacco, R., Parillo, M., Rivellese, A.A., Lasorella, G., Giacco, A., D'Episcopo, L., and Riccardi, G. (2000) Long-term dietary treatment with increased amounts at fiber-rich low-glycemic index natural foods improves blood glucose control and reduces the number of hypoglycemic events in type 1 diabetic patients . Diabetes Care , 23 : 1461 – 1466 .

14. Hangen , L. , and Bennink , M.R. (2002) Consumption of black beans and navy beans (Phaseolus vulgaris) reduced azoxymethane-induced colon cancer in rats . Nutrition and Cancer , 44 : 60 – 65 . He , J.A. , and Giusti, M.M. (2010) Anthocyanins: natural colorants with health-promoting properties . Annual Review of Food Science and Technology , 1 : 163 – 186

15. Jeng, T.L., Shih, Y.J., Lai, C.C., Wu, M.T., and Sung, J.M. (2010) Anti-oxidative characterisation of NaN3-induced common bean mutants . Food Chemistry , 119 : 1006 – 1011.

16. Kanaya, K., Tada, S., Mori, B., Takahashi , R., Ikegami, S., Kurasawa, S., Okuzaki, M., Mori, Y., and Innami, S. (2007) A simplified modification of the AOAC official method for determination of total dietary fiber using

newly developed enzymes: preliminary interlaboratory study . Journal of AOAC International , 90 : 225 – 237.

17. Koleckar, V., Kubikova, K., Rehakova, Z., Kuca, K., Jun, D., Jahodar, L., and Opletal , L. (2008) Condensed and hydrolysable tannins as antioxidants influencing the health . Mini Reviews in Medicinal Chemistry , 8 : 436 – 447 .

18. Le Berre-Anton, V., Bompard-Gilles, C., Payan , F., and Rouge, P. (1997) Characterization and functional properties of the alpha-amylase inhibitor (alpha-AI) from kidney bean (Phaseolus vulgaris) seeds . Biochimica Et Biophysica Acta-Protein Structure and Molecular Enzymology , 1343 : 31 – 40 .

19. Marko, A.J., Miller, R.A., Kelman , A., and Frauwirth , K.A. (2010) Induction of glucose metabolism in stimulated T lymphocytes is regulated by mitogen-activated protein kinase signaling. PLoS One, 5 : e15425.

20. Nothlings, U., Murphy, S.P., Wilkens, L.R. , Henderson , B.E., and Kolonel, L.N. (2007) Flavonols and pancreatic cancer risk - The multiethnic cohort study . American Journal of Epidemiology , 166 : 924 – 931 .

21. Okada , Y. , Okada , M. , and Sagesaka , Y. (2010) Screening of dried plant seed extracts for adiponectin production activity and tumor necrosis factor-alpha inhibitory activity on 3 T3-L1 adipocytes . Plant Foods for Human Nutrition , 65 : 225 – 232 .

22. Reed, J.D. (1995) Nutritional toxicology of tannins and related polyphenols in forage legumes. Journal of Animal Science , 73 : 1516 – 1528 .

23. Tormo, M.A., Gil-Exojo, I., Romero de Tejada, A., and Campillo, J.E. (2006) White bean amylase inhibitor administered orally reduces glycaemia in type 2 diabetic rats . The British Journal of Nutrition , 96 : 539 – 544 . Slavin, J., and Jacobs, D.R. (2010) Dietary fiber: all

fibers are not alike. In Wilson, T. (ed.), Nutrition guide for physicians (pp. 13–24). Totowa, N.J.: Humana .

24. Udani, J., and Singh, B.B. (2007) Blocking carbohydrate absorption and weight loss: a clinical trial using a proprietary fractionated white bean extract . Alternative Therapies in Health and Medicine , 13 : 32 – 37

25. U.S. Department of Agriculture, Agricultural Research Service . (2010) USDA National Nutrient Database for Standard Reference, Release 23. Nutrient Data Laboratory Home Page, http://www.ars.usda.gov/ba/ bhnrc/ndl. Vásquez-Arroyo, J., Sessitsch, A., Martinez, E., and Pena-Cabriales, J.J. (1998) Nitrogen fixation and nodule occupancy by native strains of Rhizobium on different cultivars of common bean (Phaseolus vulgaris L.) . Plant and Soil , 204 : 147 – 154

26. Woodman, O.L., and Chan, E.C. (2004) Vascular and anti-oxidant actions of flavonols and flavones . Clinical and Experimental Pharmacology and Physiology , 31 : 786 – 790 . Yang , S.S., Valdes-Lopez , O., Xu , W.W. , Bucciarelli , B., Gronwald, J.W., Hernandez, G., and Vance, C.P. (2010) Transcript profiling of common bean (Phaseolus vulgaris L.) using the GeneChip Soybean Genome Array: optimizing analysis by masking biased probes . BMC Plant Biology, 10 : 85 .

Chapter-12

The Nutraceutical Properties and Health Benefits of Pseudocereals

Introduction

Since ancient times, cereals like wheat, rice, and corn have been recognized for their crucial role in meeting societal food demands, constituting approximately 80% of food consumption. Efforts to enhance their nutritional value involve biofortification, a process where their micronutrient content is increased through selective breeding, genetic modification, or enriched fertilizers to bolster their nutritional profile with essential vitamins and other micronutrients.

In contrast, pseudocereals, while naturally rich in these essential micronutrients, remain largely unexplored for consumption and large-scale production. These pseudocereals can serve as abundant alternatives to traditional cereals. Unlike true cereals, which originate from grasses, pseudocereals belong to non-grasses. Their kernels can be ground into flour and utilized similarly to cereals. Botanically, pseudocereals are dicotyledonous, differing from the monocotyledonous nature of cereals.

Numerous pseudocereals are currently undergoing research and widespread cultivation, including Chia (Salvia hispanica), Quinoa (Chenopodium quinoa), Buckwheat (Fagopyrum spp.), and Amaranth (Amaranthus spp.). These varieties hold promise for their nutritional benefits and versatile culinary applications (Figure 1).

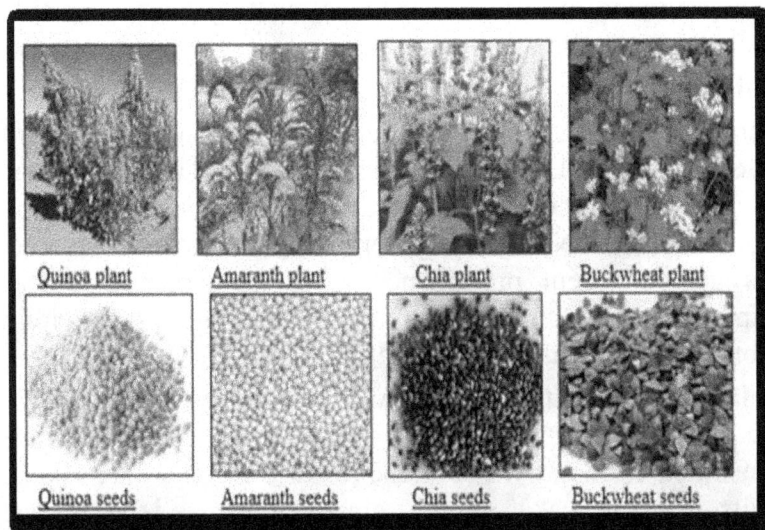

| Quinoa plant | Amaranth plant | Chia plant | Buckwheat plant |
| Quinoa seeds | Amaranth seeds | Chia seeds | Buckwheat seeds |

Figure 1: Different types of pseudo cereals

Pseudocereals boast a rich array of bioactive compounds, including amino acids, antioxidants, flavonoids, polyphenols, minerals, vitamins, lignans, dietary fiber, unsaturated fatty acids, and other vital constituents. They are considered potential alternatives to cereals and other food sources, particularly in regions lacking protein sources and facing socioeconomic challenges related to insufficient food production.

In terms of safety, pseudocereals present lower levels of anti-nutritional factors and intrinsic toxins, such as saponins, which are typically found in smaller amounts. Saponins, known for their potential negative impact on the intestinal tract, are absorbed in limited quantities when consuming pseudocereals. For instance, amaranth seeds exhibit relatively low saponin content (0.09%), resulting in reduced toxicity compared to certain cereals.

Ecologically, the utilization of pseudocereals contributes to enhancing natural resource diversity and abundance. Their adoption is recognized for their functional, social, ecological, economic, and nutritional attributes, making them adaptable to challenging climatic conditions.

Chia

Chia (Salvia hispanica) is an annual flowering plant belonging to the Lamiaceae, or mint, family. The term "chia" originates from the Nahuatl word "chian," meaning oily. This crop, native to Northern Guatemala and Southern Mexico, has gained recent prominence in South America and is primarily cultivated in mountainous regions within subtropical and temperate climates.

Chia offers versatile uses, available in mucilage, whole seeds, seed oil, and flour forms. These seeds can be consumed on their own or added to various foods like salads, fruits, yogurts, cakes, bread, granola bars, and beverages. Renowned for their substantial fiber content, omega-3 fatty acids, proteins, essential minerals, and antioxidants, chia seeds are believed to enhance digestive health, elevate omega-3 fatty acid levels in the blood, and mitigate risk factors associated with heart disease and diabetes.

The seeds are esteemed for their richness in dietary fiber, fats, minerals, polyphenolic compounds, and protein. Chia oil, particularly noted for its polyunsaturated fatty acids (PUFA), is highly regarded. Studies emphasize its exceptional composition, boasting higher levels of alpha-linolenic acid (ALA) and omega-3 fatty acids compared to other natural sources.

Chia has become a pivotal ingredient in producing functional food products globally due to its balanced blend of bioactive components. Its consumption is linked to a range of health benefits associated with chronic diseases such as cardiovascular diseases, obesity, cancer, and diabetes, contributing to the increasing utilization of chia over the years.

Quinoa

Quinoa (Chenopodium quinoa) is an annual, dicotyledonous, and self-pollinating plant belonging to the Chenopodiaceae family. Botanically akin to amaranth and spinach, quinoa is classified as a pseudocereal and is distinct from grasses. Originating from South America's Andean region, particularly Peru, Ecuador, and Bolivia, quinoa is prized for its salt and drought tolerance, as well as its resilience in barren and cold environments.

Cultivated primarily for its edible seeds, quinoa's seeds are small, round, and flattened, measuring about 1.5 mm in diameter. These seeds are rich in dietary fiber, proteins, minerals, fatty acids, and the vitamin B complex. Additionally, quinoa harbors an extensive array of bioactive compounds like polyphenols, flavonoids, and saponins, surpassing many other grain crops in their abundance (Alan, 2011).

Recognized by the United Nations Food and Agriculture Organization (UNFAO) as a plant that fulfills fundamental nutritional needs, quinoa has been referred to as "the mother of grain" by ancient Incan civilization. Research indicates that quinoa seeds possess higher biological value—a measure of retained protein for growth and maintenance—compared to other cereal grains. Specifically, quinoa showcases a biological value of 73%, surpassing major cereal crops like rice (56%), wheat (49%), and corn (36%). Remarkably, quinoa's protein value, ranging from 12.9% to 16.5%, even exceeds that of emblematic cereal grains.

In nutritional equivalence to meat products, quinoa's protein content makes it an exceptional dietary resource, elevating its status as a highly valuable food source.

Amaranth

The Amaranthaceae family, often known as the "Amaranth family," derives its name from the Greek word "Anthos," signifying longevity and unwilting, referring to the flower. Taxonomically, this family is divided into two sections: Blitopsis dumort and Amaranthus saucer, each comprising nearly an equal number of species.

Amaranth grows rapidly, particularly in tropical regions, making it a cost-effective dark green vegetable with a relatively low production cost. These attributes have earned it the moniker "poor man's vegetable." Widely found in temperate, tropical, and subtropical regions globally, amaranth is typically harvested during the summer months when other green vegetables are scarce in the market.

Highly recommended as both a grain crop and a vegetable, amaranth serves as an economical nutrient source, especially rich in protein, catering to the dietary needs of underserved populations in developing countries. This plant holds significant nutritional value, providing a noteworthy amount of carbohydrates, proteins, fats, dietary fiber, and various micronutrients.

Amaranth is unique as its seeds are utilized as a cereal, while its leaves are commonly consumed as a vegetable. The versatility of Amaranthus extends to its usage in various food products, including pancakes, noodles, pasta, biscuits, candies, and cookies, showcasing its adaptability in diverse culinary applications.

Buckwheat

Buckwheat, classified under the Polygonaceae family, serves as an alternative and cover crop, offering grain-like seeds often associated with cereal groups despite its botanical distinction. Two primary types, tartary (green buckwheat, Fagopyrum tataricum) and common (Fagopyrum esculentum), are globally cultivated and consumed. Despite its name, buckwheat shares no botanical relationship with wheat as it belongs to the sorrel, rhubarb, and knotweed family, rather than being a grass.

Prominent countries such as China, USA, Russia, Canada, Germany, France, Poland, and Italy engage in extensive buckwheat cultivation. Renowned for its balanced nutritional profile, buckwheat seeds, although slightly less digestible, serve as a pseudocereal due to their complex carbohydrate structure, making them adaptable for culinary purposes akin to cereals.

The buckwheat plant stands as a substantial nutritive resource for both animals and humans, offering protein, carbohydrates, dietary fibers, and a notable concentration of B vitamins, minerals, essential amino acids, and antioxidants, surpassing many traditional cereals. Despite the presence of anti-nutritive factors and lower digestibility attributed to its high fiber content, buckwheat remains valuable, providing essential nutrients for animal and human health.

Acknowledged as a viable alternative to other cereal crops, buckwheat's adaptability to harsh climatic conditions positions it as a favorable choice in human diets and animal feed, demonstrating its potential versatility across various environments.

Prevention of chronic diseases by using pseudocereals

The shifting global dietary patterns towards energy-dense, low unprocessed carbohydrate, high-fat diets have contributed to the rise of chronic non-communicable diseases (NCDs) such as atherosclerosis, diabetes, heart issues, stroke, hypertension, certain cancers, and obesity. These diseases are becoming prominent causes of vulnerability and premature mortality in both developed and developing nations. In response, the exploration of new functional food sources that possess properties counteracting these ailments is gaining attention. Several in vivo studies have been conducted to assess the potential of pseudocereals in preventing chronic diseases. Figure 2 presents a schematic representation summarizing the health benefits associated with pseudocereal consumption.

Chia seeds, utilized as flour or whole grains, are integrated into various products like salads, yogurts, beverages, and bread. The bioactive compounds within chia seeds have attracted considerable research interest due to their potential against infectious diseases like CVDs, obesity, cancer, and diabetes. Research highlights the significant fiber, iron, omega-3 fatty acid, calcium, and magnesium content in chia seeds, surpassing even milk in certain nutrients. Evidence suggests that regular intake of chia seeds aids in stabilizing blood glucose levels in diabetic patients, curbing platelet aggregation to prevent strokes and heart attacks, and reducing systolic blood pressure by up to 6 mmHg.

Numerous investigations have explored the health benefits of quinoa. Daily consumption of quinoa has shown promise in reducing cardiovascular risks, blood fat and glucose levels, enhancing plasma antioxidant activity, and minimizing systemic inflammation in at-risk individuals. Studies on a quinoa-based diet revealed decreases in vitamin E, thiobarbituric acid reactive substances (TBARS), serum triglyceride concentrations, and an increase in enterolignans excretion through urine. Notably, it led to an increase in glutathione (GSH) and a decrease in total LDL cholesterol (LDL-c), indicating a favorable impact on health. Additionally, even minor changes in body mass index (BMI), body mass, and circulating lipid levels resulting from consuming quinoa biscuits contribute to reducing CVD risks in older adults.

Coronary artery disease (CAD) is a complex ailment associated with mortality and morbidity, often linked to the inflammatory process. Studies on Amaranthus caudatus L. demonstrated its potential anti-atherosclerotic properties in rabbits, significantly reducing major risk factors such as apolipoprotein B (apoB), oxidized low-density lipoprotein (OLDL), serum lipoproteins, and inflammatory markers, thus impeding atherosclerosis. Diets enriched with amaranth were observed to markedly reduce cholesterol, LDL cholesterol, and triglycerides in hypercholesterolemic rabbits compared to a control diet, suggesting its therapeutic potential against chronic diseases.

Antioxidant activity of pseudocereals

Studies have highlighted the antioxidant potential of chia protein hydrolysates, indicating their ability to prevent lipid oxidation and enhance the survival of yeast Saccharomyces cerevisiae when exposed to hydrogen peroxide (H_2O_2) in meat systems. Further investigations on chia papain hydrolysates demonstrated antioxidant potential along with anti-inflammatory properties during gastrointestinal digestion. These fractions exhibited inhibition of enzymes such as inducible nitric oxide synthase (iNOS) and cyclooxygenases (COX1 and COX2), indicating anti-inflammatory activity. Quinoa, known for its high-quality proteins containing all essential amino acids, has shown promising bioactive potential, particularly its protein hydrolysates. Recent research has unveiled quinoa proteins' anti-diabetic potential by inhibiting enzymes like α-amylase, α-glucosidase, and dipeptidyl peptidase-IV, along with antiproliferative and antioxidative effects on colon tumor cells.

Amaranth has also demonstrated antioxidant effects, especially in its grain form. Hydrolysates of amaranth peptides showed resistance against dipeptidyl peptidase-IV, inhibition of angiotensin-altering enzymes, and antioxidant properties. Animal studies with amaranth seed extract (ASE) indicated substantial hepatoprotective potential, particularly at a dose of 400 mg/kg, increasing the activities of antioxidative enzymes like superoxide dismutase (SOD) and catalase, thus showcasing its antioxidant capacity.

Research exploring the antioxidant properties of buckwheat has shown an increase in antioxidant potential in the blood of subjects after consuming buckwheat. Studies assessing buckwheat protein hydrolysates revealed strong antioxidant activities in vitro.

Both amaranth and quinoa seeds are recognized as rich sources of antioxidants. Their antioxidant potential, measured through various assays like DPPH, ORAC, and FRAP, correlated positively with their total phenolic content (TPC). Lipophilic antioxidants in these seeds, including tocopherols, fatty acids, and carotenoids, contribute to their antioxidant activity. Quinoa seeds, in particular, exhibited higher antioxidant activities compared to amaranth seeds, attributed to their higher total carotenoid index (TCI), unsaturated fatty acids (UFAs), and total tocopherol index (TTI). These antioxidants play a crucial role in counteracting oxidative stress caused by an imbalance between reactive oxygen species (ROS) formation and antioxidant defense mechanisms

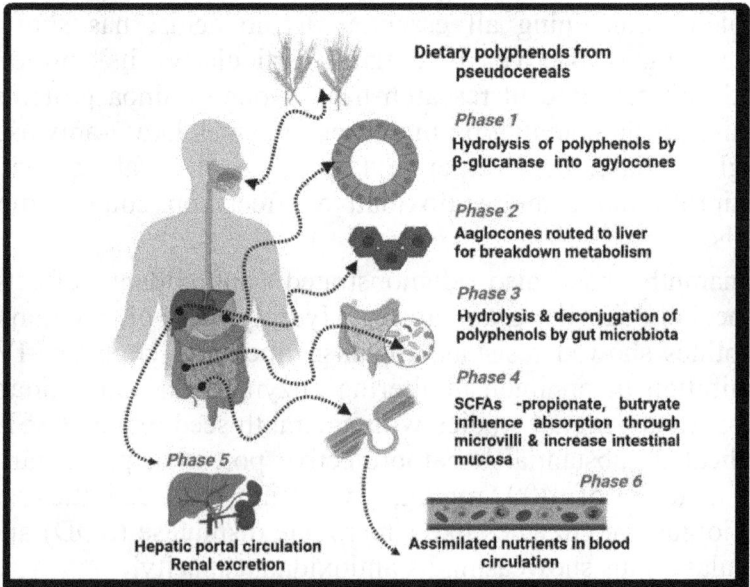

Figure 3 : The role of dietary polyphenols of pseudocereals in human health maintenance

Hypolipidemic effects of pseudocereals

Research has outlined the role of phytochemicals found in pseudocereals in managing hypolipidemia. Protein hydrolysates derived from chia by-products have been identified as potential hypocholesterolemic agents suitable for incorporation into functional foods and nutraceuticals, presenting promising avenues for human health and food safety. Additionally, a study focused on chia seeds explored their impact on plasma triglyceride levels in healthy individuals with mildly elevated lipid levels. The findings suggested that chia could serve as a safe alternative therapy with clinical significance for primary prevention of cardiovascular diseases (CVDs) by regulating undesirable cholesterol levels. Another recent study indicated that chia intake could prevent or mitigate hepatitis while reducing cholesterol levels in rats. The high content of phenolic compounds and omega-3 fatty acids, specifically alpha-linolenic acid (ALA), contributes to the hypolipidemic and hepatoprotective effects associated with chia.

Studies investigating the effects of quinoa seed powder (QSP) on male rats examined its potential in mitigating hypercholesterolemia. The in vivo study revealed that a diet enriched with QSP not only improved weight gain and feed consumption but also reduced lipid profiles and the risk to organ function. These findings suggest that QSP could mitigate the adverse effects of hypercholesterolemia. Additionally, recent research has highlighted the cholesterol-lowering effects of quinoa yogurt.

It's believed that atherosclerosis, a condition stemming from severe inflammation, involves arterial thickening due to plaque buildup, primarily cholesterol. Pseudocereals exhibit hypolipidemic effects that help reduce the risk of atherosclerosis. Studies have examined amaranth's anti-atherosclerotic action in rabbits induced with hypercho-lesterolemia, noting reductions in LDL and triglyceride concentrations. The hydrolysis of Amaranthus cruentus yielded binding peptides that were evaluated for their impact on the enzyme HMG-CoA reductase, crucial in cholesterol biosynthesis.

In assessing the physiological properties of buckwheat flour, particularly its high protein content, researchers investigated its effects on gallstone formation, blood cholesterol, and body fat in mice. The results indicated its significant potential against hypercholesterolemia, gallstones, and obesity, positioning it as an effective remedy for these conditions. Additionally, a study focusing on hyperlipidemic rats analyzed the lipid profile and antioxidation status following supplementation with Tartary buckwheat bran extract (green buckwheat). The extract notably reduced serum triglycerides and cholesterol levels in rats while enhancing serum antioxidant capacity and inhibiting lipid peroxide formation.

Hypoglycemic effects of pseudocereals

In rat studies, regular chia consumption demonstrated enhanced digestibility, lowered cholesterol, improved glycemic profiles, and reduced liver fat, leading to improved intestinal tissue function. Gazem, Puneeth, and Sharada (2016) highlighted chia seed oil's antidiabetic, hypolipidemic, and anti-proliferative properties. Investigating the potential anti-diabetic effects of amaranth grain and oil in rats induced with streptozotocin-induced diabetes, Kim et al. (2006) found that supplementation with amaranth grain and oil increased serum insulin levels and decreased serum glucose levels in diabetic rats.

Quinoa proteins are recognized for their potential in developing functional foods and nutraceuticals to manage diabetes. Studies emphasize that firm glycemic control can reduce the risk of severe diabetic complications, and a low glycemic index diet can improve insulin resistance and glycemia in type-2 diabetes mellitus (T2DM). Gabrial, Shakib, and Gabrial (2016) investigated the effects of quinoa and buckwheat-based breakfasts on glucose fluctuations in both healthy and diabetic subjects. Their in vivo study revealed that pseudocereal-based breakfasts have the potential to stabilize blood glucose levels, suggesting their beneficial inclusion in the daily diet plans of diabetic individuals for a healthier life .

Anti-cancer effects of pseudocereals

In recent findings, chia seeds have emerged as a rich source of phytosterols, exhibiting preventive qualities against cardiovascular diseases (CVDs) and demonstrating antimicrobial, antioxidant, and potential anticancer properties. A study delved into the anti-cancer and anti-inflammatory attributes of chia seeds, assessing their anti-lipoxygenase (LO) activity. The outcomes indicated that chia seed oil (CSO), used alone or in conjunction with vegetable oil, serves as a cooperative and suitable dietary supplement. Supplementation of CSO was found effective in staving off or delaying the onset of severe modern lifestyle-related ailments.

Amaranthus species showcase robust antioxidant, lectin, and anti-proliferative activities specifically on EAC cells, primarily through mitochondrial-mediated apoptosis. Studies also noted the antitumor properties exhibited by A. mantegazzianus seeds.

In the realm of buckwheat cultivation in vast regions of Northwest China, both tartary and common buckwheat varieties stand out as reservoirs of bioactive compounds. Ethanolic extracts of buckwheat were explored for their protective effects against DNA damage and antioxidant potential. Findings revealed the significant potential of buckwheat extracts in preventing DNA damage caused by hydroxy radicals, attributed to their radical scavenging and iron-chelating activities. Additionally, a peptide (AQCGAQGGGATCPGG) found in buckwheat exhibited antiproliferative properties against certain cancer cell types like breast cancer, leukemia, and hepatoma, along with demonstrating antifungal characteristics.

Hypotensive effects of pseudocereals

Orona-Tamayo and colleagues (2015) highlighted the sudden surge in chia's inclusion in human diets, attributing it to its antioxidant properties and its impact on reducing hypertension. Similar findings were documented by Segura-Campos et al. (2013), emphasizing the antihypertensive effects of chia. Buckwheat, too, has shown promise in reducing blood pressure, supported by several studies showcasing its antihypertensive activities.

Quinoa proteins harbor a significant concentration of bioactive peptides. In a study utilizing simulated gastrointestinal digestion, quinoa protein hydrolysates exhibited notable potential in hypertension management. Consequently, quinoa protein becomes a potential ingredient for developing functional foods aimed at controlling blood pressure. Assessing the angiotensin-I converting enzyme (ACE) inhibition activity of various cereals and pseudocereals revealed quinoa and buckwheat as leaders, with ACE inhibition activities of 23.3% and 22.8%, respectively. Amaranth displayed lower inhibition activity compared to quinoa at 8.8%, yet higher than major cereals like wheat and rice. Studies in hypertensive rats indicate that quinoa consumption led to a reduction in systolic blood pressure, indicating its richness in beneficial minerals. Given the array of bioactive compounds in quinoa, the creation of functional foods utilizing quinoa protein hydrolysates with antioxidant and antihypertensive properties is feasible.

Angiotensin-I converting enzyme is pivotal in blood pressure and cardiovascular function regulation. Numerous studies have underscored the antihypertensive activity of A. hypochondriacus. Amaranth and quinoa have been recognized for their allergenicity, antihypertensive, and antioxidative activities, backed by multiple research works. Additionally, A. mantegazzianus contains encrypted peptides released through hydrolysis, showcasing antihypertensive activity.

Hepatoprotective effects of pseudocereals

The hepatoprotective and antioxidant properties of the ethanolic extract of A. spinosus (ASE) were examined in rats with liver damage induced by CCl4. The results strongly supported the protective capacity of A. spinosus extract against CCl4-induced liver damage in the studied animals. This investigation suggested that the presence of phenolic compounds and flavonoids in ASE might account for its hepatoprotective activity. Similarly, another study highlighted the potent antioxidative and hepatoprotective effects of the ethanolic seed extract of A. hypochondriacus in rats treated with sodium arsenite. The effectiveness of the ethanol extract of A. hypochondriacus showed dose dependency and exhibited higher activity compared to the control group at 300 mg/kg b.w.

In rats, methanolic extracts of the entire A. caudatus plant displayed hepatoprotective potential. Furthermore, research focusing on tartary buckwheat extract (TBE) enriched with D-ChiroInositol (DCI) showcased its defensive abilities against liver injury and hyperglycemia induced by a high fructose diet in rats. These findings suggested that TBE consumption could serve as a viable protective or therapeutic approach for hepatic steatosis, oxidative damage, and hyperglycemia stemming from a high-fat diet. Quinoa seeds also exhibited hepatoprotective potential in certain studies. In vivo investigations in mice demonstrated the seeds' ability to protect against liver injury induced by CCl4. Additionally, a study highlighted the considerable effects of artichoke extract on CCl4-induced liver damage, emphasizing the plant's hepatoprotective potential. Figure 5 delineates the interconnectedness within the gut-liver axis regulated by bioactive compounds found in pseudocereals.

Anti-inflammatory properties of pseudocereals

Quinoa polyphenols have been observed to reduce interleukin-8 (IL-8), interleukin-1 (IL-1), and tumor necrosis factor (TNF) cytokines in cultured colonic epithelial Caco-2 cells. This action inhibits inflammation and supports gastrointestinal health in experimental mice. In a study involving overweight postmenopausal women, consuming quinoa flakes for 28 days led to a reduction in interleukin-6 (IL-6) levels, unlike those consuming corn flakes. Since IL-6 is a pro-inflammatory marker, the decrease in its plasma expression due to quinoa consumption suggests a potential means of managing inflammation in postmenopausal women. Quinoa seed saponins have also been associated with reducing the overproduction of inflammatory cytokines, including IL-6, TNF, and nitric oxide (NO), indicating the potential use of quinoa saponins as a functional food compound for preventing and managing inflammation.

Research by Tang et al. (2015) highlighted that the polyunsaturated fatty acids (PUFA) and phenolics found in cooked quinoa significantly reduced the production of the pro-inflammatory factor IL-8. They also downregulated the messenger ribonucleic acid (mRNA) expression of IL-8, IL-6, TNF, COX-2, and IL-1 while up-regulating mRNA expression of the anti-inflammatory cytokine IL-10, and this effect was dosage-dependent.

In an experimental mouse model, a single oral dose of hydromethanolic extract from amaranth seeds increased the concentration of nitrite ($NO2-$) and nitrate ($NO3-$) while reducing the production of nitric oxide (NO) in a mouse macrophage-like cell line known as RAW264.7. Betacyanins and selenium present in the edible seeds of amaranth sprouts were found to hinder the translocation of nuclear factor kappa B (NF-κB) to the nucleus, displaying anti-inflammatory actions by significantly reducing pro-inflammatory markers like IL-6 in RAW 264.7 macrophages.

Prevention of polycystic ovary syndrome (PCOS) by pseudocereals

Polycystic Ovary Syndrome (PCOS) is a hormonal disorder characterized by significant insulin resistance, anovulation, and elevated androgen levels. Women affected by PCOS are at a higher risk of developing type 2 diabetes mellitus. There's been limited research exploring the impact of pseudocereals on preventing PCOS. Studies have highlighted fagopyritols, specific bioactive compounds found in buckwheat and categorized as soluble carbohydrates, which exhibit promising effects in addressing PCOS and type 2 diabetes. Fagopyritols have garnered significant interest due to their potential in this regard. However, research findings suggest that while buckwheat may not directly prevent PCOS, it could potentially play an indirect role in its prevention.

Pseudocereals as skin curative

In recent times, there's been a surge in the popularity of natural beauty products crafted from plant-based ingredients, owing to the active components present in plant proteins and their minimal side effects. However, there's still a lack of comprehensive research exploring the potential of pseudocereals in skincare. A study conducted by Jeong et al. (2010) investigated the effects of topical application of omega-3 fatty acids derived from chia oil formulations. The results revealed significant improvements in skin hydration, chronic prurigo nodularis, and lichen simplex in all subjects, suggesting chia oil's potential as a skin healing agent.

Quinoa protein is recognized as an exceptional raw material

utilized in cosmetics. Its hydrolysates serve as beneficial agents for skin nourishment and natural hair conditioning. Additionally, quinoa's saponins act as natural plant-based surfactants. Quinoa seed oil, consumed for therapeutic purposes, contains various mineral elements that hold promise as nutritional components for human skin. Moreover, the amino acids and vitamins present in quinoa offer potential for formulating diverse skincare products and cosmetics.

Suggestions and future perspectives

The economic potential of pseudocereals remains largely unexplored, warranting further research to realize their full benefits. Incorporating pseudocereals into our staple diets, either independently or in conjunction with traditional cereals, holds promise for improving life quality by supplying essential nutrients that reduce oxidative stress and, consequently, enhance life expectancy.

There's a pressing need to adopt an industrial approach toward pseudocereals, with ample room for exploration. Developing value-added products on an industrial scale presents an opportunity to address nutrient-related malnutrition, even in developed nations where diets often emphasize caloric density. This exploration could pave the way for new markets and innovative nutritional solutions.

References

1. Adebowale, O. J., and O. O Ajibode. 2022. Fortification of cassava starch with coconut residue: effects on flours' functional properties and products' (Tapioca meals) nutritional and sensory qualities. Natural Resources for Human Health 2(2):200–207.
2. Ahmad, I., Rashid M. H. U., Nawaz, S., Asif M., Farooq T. H., Shahbaz Z., M. Kashif, M. Shaheen. 2022. Effect of

different compost concentrations on the growth yield of Bombax Ceiba (Simal). Natural Resources for Human Health 2(2):222–227.

3. Ahmed, J., L. Thomas, Y. A. Arfat, and A. Joseph. 2018. Rheological, structural and functional properties of high-pressure treated quinoa starch in dispersions. Carbohydrate Polymers 197:649–57. doi: 10.1016/j.carbpol.2018.05.081.

4. Alan, B. 2011. Quinoa, an ancient crop to contribute to world food security. In 37th FAO Conference. Alghamdi, E. S. 2018. Protective effect of quinoa (Chenopodium quinoa willd.) seeds against hypercholesterolemia in male rats. Pharmacophore 9 (6):11–21.

5. Barrio, D. A., and M. C. Añón. 2010. Potential antitumor properties of a protein isolate obtained from the seeds of Amaranthus mantegazzianus. European Journal of Nutrition 49 (2):73–82.

6. Bojňanská, T., H. Frančáková, P. Chlebo, and A. Vollmannová. 2009. Rutin content in buckwheat enriched bread and influence of its consumption on plasma total antioxidant status. Czech Journal of Food Sciences 27 (Special Issue 1):S236–S240. doi: 10.17221/967-CJFS.

7. Carrasco, E, and J. L. Soto. 2010. Importancia de los granos andinos. In Granos andinos: avances, logros y experiencias desarrolladas en quinua, canihua y kiwicha en Per u, eds. R. Bravo, R. Valdivia, K. Andrade, S. Paludosi, and M. Jagger, 6–10. Rome, Italy: Biodiversity International. Carvalho, A., J. Marchini, and A. Navarro. 2015. Quinoa or corn flakes to prevent peripheral inflammation after menopause? Journal of Obesity & Eating Disorders 1:4.

8. De Carvalho, F. G., P. P. Ovídio, G. J. Padovan, A. A. Jordão Junior, J. S. Marchini, and A. M. Navarro. 2014. Metabolic parameters of postmenopausal women after quinoa or corn flakes intake – A prospective and double-

blind study. International Journal of Food Sciences and Nutrition 65 (3):380–5.

9. Fritz, M., B. Vecchi, G. Rinaldi, and M. C. Añón. 2011. Amaranth seed protein hydrolysates have in vivo and in vitro antihypertensive activity. Food Chemistry 126 (3):878–84. doi: 10.1016/j.foodchem.2010.11.065.

10. Gabrial, S. G. N., M.-C R. Shakib, and G. N. Gabrial. 2016. Effect of pseudocereal-based breakfast meals on the first and second meal glucose tolerance in healthy and diabetic subjects. Open Access Macedonian Journal of Medical Sciences 4 (4):565–73. doi: 10.3889/oamjms.2016.115

11. Hu, Y., Y. Zhao, D. Ren, J. Guo, Y. Luo, and X. Yang. 2015. Hypoglycemic and hepatoprotective effects of d-chiro-inositol-enriched tartary buckwheat extract in high fructose-fed mice. Food & Function 6 (12):3760–9. doi: 10.1039/C5FO00612K.

12. Ixtaina, V. Y., S. M. Nolasco, and M. C. Tom. 2008. Physical properties of chia (Salvia hispanica L.) seeds. Industrial Crops and Products 28 (3):286–93. doi: 10.1016/j.indcrop.2008.03.009.

13. Liberal, Â., R. C. Calhelha, C. Pereira, F. Adega, L. Barros, M. Dueñas, C. Santos-Buelga, R. M. V. Abreu, and I. C. F. R. Ferreira. 2016. A comparison of the bioactivity and phytochemical profile of three different cultivars of globe amaranth: Red, white, and pink. Food & Function 7 (2):679–88.

14. Pamela, E. A. I., A. O. Oyeronke, A. G. Michael, O. A. Ayodeji, A. O. Solomon, and M. A. Ayodeji. 2015. Hepatoprotective effect of Amaranthus hypochondriacus seed extract on sodium arsenite-induced toxicity in male Wistar rats. Journal of Medicinal Plants Research 9 (26):731–40. doi: 10.5897/JMPR2015.5860.

15. Paweł, P., B. Henryk, Z. Paweł, G. Shela, F. Maria, and Z. Zofia. 2009. Anthocyanins, total polyphenols and

antioxidant activity in amaranth and quinoa seeds and sprouts during their growth. Food Chemistry 115:994–8

16. Vuksan, V., D. Whitham, J. L. Sievenpiper, A. L. Jenkins, A. L. Rogovik, R. P. Bazinet, E. Vidgen, and A. Hanna. 2007. Supplementation of conventional therapy with the novel grain Salba (Salvia hispanica L.) improves major and emerging cardiovascular risk factors in type 2 diabetes. Diabetes Care 30 (11):2804–10. doi: 10.2337/dc07-1144.

17. Wang, M., J. R. Liu, J. M. Gao, J. W. Parry, and Y. M. Wei. 2009. Antioxidant activity of Tartary buckwheat bran extract and its effect on the lipid profile of hyperlipidemic rats. Journal of Agricultural and Food Chemistry 57 (11):5106–12. doi: 10.1021/jf900194s

18. Zeashan, H., G. Amresh, S. Singh, and C. V. Rao. 2008. Hepatoprotective activity of Amaranthus spinosus in experimental animals. Food and Chemical Toxicology: An International Journal Published for the British Industrial Biological Research Association 46 (11):3417–21.

Chapter-13

An Overview of Herbal Nutraceuticals and their Therapeutic Effect

Introduction

Nutraceuticals, derived from food sources, encompass a range of products including dietary supplements, herbal items, genetically modified foods, and vitamins. Rich in bioactive compounds, they provide health benefits and nutritional value, aiding in disease prevention and treatment. Herbal nutraceuticals, derived from plants and their parts like oils, roots, seeds, and berries, support overall wellness and address various acute and chronic health issues linked to poor dietary habits. Across ancient cultures like those in India and China, herbal remedies have been deeply ingrained, serving both as sustenance and medicinal aids. Today, the field of nutraceuticals has evolved into a specialized scientific industry, with products backed by rigorous data, ongoing research, and advancements in technology to ensure their effectiveness and safety.

Sources of Bioactive Compounds (Herbs)

Aloe Vera

Aloe vera, scientifically labeled Aloe barbadensis Miller, is a succulent plant commonly grown as a household plant. It serves as a natural remedy for minor skin irritations like sunburns and wounds. Beyond that, it finds application in managing acne, soothing symptoms of dermatitis, easing mild stomach discomfort, and supporting hair growth. Its composition includes various bioactive elements such as flavonoids, lectins, terpenoids, fatty acids, tannins, anthraquinones, pectins, hemicelluloses, glucomannan, campesterol, β-sitosterol, salicylic acid, and an array of vitamins like A, C, E, β-carotene, B1, B2, B3, B6, choline,

172

B12, and folic acid. These diverse compounds demonstrate effectiveness in various realms including anti-hyperlipidemic, anticancer, anti-diabetic, anti-mutagenic, anti-inflammatory, and antioxidant properties. Notably, recent research highlights aloe-emodin, an anthraquinone extracted from aloe vera leaf, showcasing significant anti-leukemic effects on lymphoblastic leukemia cells compared to standard clinical drugs. Additionally, investigations by Huseini et al. suggest that aloe vera gel exhibits potential as an anti-hyperglycemic and anti-hypercholesterolemic agent, displaying positive impacts on blood glucose and lipid levels in antidiabetic evaluations.

Angelica

Angelica, scientifically termed Angelica archangelica, has enjoyed a long history as both a spice and a medicinal plant, tracing back to the 12th century. Its fruits, stems, and roots have garnered recognition for their positive impacts on human health. The bioactive constituents found in Angelica, particularly in its roots, encompass β-phellandrene, umbelliprenin, phenols, and furocoumarins like bergapten, xanthotoxin, and angelicin. This herb is utilized in the treatment of various conditions including arthritis, heartburn, flatulence, anorexia, circulation issues, respiratory catarrh, insomnia, nervousness, and plague.

Anise

Anise, scientifically referred to as Pimpinella anisum, holds a prominent place as a medicinal herb in various medical traditions, including traditional, folk, and modern pharmaceutical practices. Renowned for its licorice-like taste, anise is utilized in diverse forms such as whole, dried, and crushed, serving as a flavor enhancer and aiding in digestion. Its bioactive components include trans-anethole, coumarins like umbelliferone and bergapten, scopoletin, flavonoids such as flavonol, flavone glycosides like rutin, isoorientin, isovitexin, as well as lipids like fatty acids, beta-amyrin, stigmasterol, and their salts. Numerous studies underscore the potential benefits of anise, suggesting its efficacy in addressing issues like constipation, indigestion, menopausal symptoms, and migraines. Furthermore, research has highlighted its antioxidant, antifungal, anti-inflammatory, antibacterial, anticonvulsant, gastro-protective, anti-diabetic, analgesic, and antiviral properties.

Aralia

Aralia, scientifically termed as Polyscias fruticosa, holds a significant place in traditional medicine across Asia and the Americas. Another variety, American spikenard root or Aralia racemosa, is native to the eastern United States and is widely utilized in balsamic teas and tonics. Similar to ginseng, aralia root is believed to offer various health benefits. Poultices made from American spikenard are used to alleviate conditions like rheumatism and eczema. These species contain diverse bioactive compounds such as petroselinic acid, triterpenoid saponins, sterols, diterpenoids, and acetylenic lipids, which are employed in treating conditions like hepatitis, bruises, carbuncles, and lumps.

Bay

Bay, also known as laurel leaf or sweet bay, originates from the Mediterranean region and is prevalent in warm climates. Scientifically identified as Laurus nobilis. L., bay finds common usage in various cuisines such as French, Spanish, Italian, and Creole dishes, including soups, stews, sauces, and pickling brines. Its bioactive components encompass cholesteric-7-en-3β-ol, cholesteric-4-en-3β,6β-diol, batilol, and ceramide. This medicinal plant has been linked to reducing uric acid levels and controlling blood cholesterol. Several studies have indicated the anti-inflammatory, antidiarrheal, and anti-diabetic potential of bay leaf extracts.

Bayberry

Bayberry, recognized for its medicinal properties, contains diverse bioactive components like anthocyanidins—delphinidin–hexoside, cyanidin-3-O-galactoside, cyanidin-3-O-glucoside, pelargonidin-3-O-glucoside, and peonidin-3-O-glucoside, as well as flavonols such as myricetin-3-O-rhamnoside, myricetin deoxyhexoside–gallate, quercetin-3-O-galactoside, quercetin-3-O-glucoside, quercetin-3-O-rhamnoside, kaempferol-3-O-galactoside, and kaempferol-3-O-glucoside. Its applications span the treatment of sore throat, colitis, wounds, ulcers, headaches, colds, nausea, diarrhea, and enhancement of systemic circulation.

Bee Balm

Scientifically known as Monarda didyma L., bee balm, part of the mint family, is referred to as Oswego tea, horsemint, or bergamot. Its diverse bioactive components include polyphenols (rosmarinic acid, caffeic acid, protocatechuic acid), flavonoids (quercitrin, rhamnocitrin, luteolin), monoterpenoid aldehyde, monoterpene glycosides, triterpenes (ursolic and oleanolic acids), sesquiterpenes, resin, tannin, and essential oils (citral-geraniol and neral, linalool, eugenol, citronellal, geraniol). Extracts demonstrate diaphoretic, antiseptic, emmenagogue, antimicrobial, antispasmodic, and anti-inflammatory properties.

Burnet

Originating from western, central, and southern Europe, as well as parts of Africa and Asia, burnet—scientifically known as Sanguisorba minor—shares a taste akin to cucumber and finds its use in salads and dressings. Its bioactive profile includes phenolic acids (like chlorogenic, ellagic, gallic, caffeic, and rosmarinic acid), flavonoids, catechin derivatives (such as catechin and epigallocatechin gallate), and neolignans. Various studies highlight its effectiveness in addressing ulcerative colitis, dysentery, diarrhea, bladder problems, hemorrhoids, phlebitis, and varicose veins.

Calamint

Native to the UK, calamint plants boast bushy characteristics with thick stems spreading from rhizomes. The leaves possess a hairy or fuzzy texture. Scientifically acknowledged as Clinopodium nepeta, it features an array of beneficial active components including dihydrocarveol, monoterpenes, dihydrocarveol acetate, 1,8-cineole, cis-carvyl acetate, and pulegone. These compounds exhibit notable antioxidant, antimicrobial, anti-ulcer, anti-inflammatory, and insecticidal properties. Notably, its monoterpene components show significant antifungal potency, particularly against Trichophyton mentagrophytes.

Caraway

An indigenous biennial plant of western Asia and Europe, scientifically termed Carum carvi, caraway is valued for its seeds and roots. The licorice-flavored seeds are commonly used in various culinary preparations like breads, soups, sauces, pickles, and sauerkraut. Caraway serves as a traditional herbal remedy for conditions such as rheumatism, eye infections, and toothaches. Its bioactive component profile comprises carvacrol, carvone, α-pinene, limonene, γ-terpinene, linalool, carvenone, and p-cymene. It acts as an expectorant, stimulant, antispasmodic agent, and aids in alleviating nausea, stomach aches, and constipation.

Chamomile

Chamomile, revered as one of the oldest medicinal herbs with historical usage dating back to ancient Greek and Roman cultures, is scientifically termed Matricaria recutita. Its bioactive components like levomenol and its oxides, apigenin, azulenes, farnesene, spathulenol, and spiroethers are widely employed to address various human ailments including hay fever, muscle spasms, inflammation, menstrual disorders, wounds, ulcers, insomnia, gastrointestinal disorders, hemorrhoids, and rheumatic pain.

Dill

An annual herb from the Anethum graveolens L. family, dill shares a genus with celery and is best consumed fresh due to its rapid loss of flavor. Known for its medicinal potential, dill houses a diverse range of bioactive components including sinapic and vanillic acids, along with rutin. Traditionally, it has been utilized to address stomach ailments, colic, hiccups, bad breath, flatulence, and hemorrhoids.

Zedoary

Zedoary Known as white turmeric, zedoary—scientifically termed Curcuma zedoaria—is a rhizomatous herb native to Indonesia and India. A staple in traditional folk medicine, it's employed to manage various conditions including menstrual disorders, vomiting, dyspepsia, fatigue, anxiety, stress, inflammation, and even cancer. Zedoary contains key bioactive components like furanodienone, zederone, demethoxycurcumin, germacrone, bisdemethoxycurcumin, 1,7-diphenyl-(4E,6E)-4,6-heptadien-3-ol, curcumin, and ar-turmerone. Studies have demonstrated its strong anti-proliferative and anti-metastatic effects on esophageal cancer TE-8 cells and its potential in inhibiting tumor formation.

Yarrow

Yarrow Scientifically named Achillea millefolium, yarrow is celebrated for its array of blossom colors and therapeutic properties. Its bioactive components encompass azulene, caryophyllene, thujone, eucalyptol, α- and β-pinene, borneol, lactones, tannins, and alkaloids. Yarrow finds application in treating hay fever, the common cold, menstrual issues, diarrhea, dysentery, loss of appetite, gastric discomfort, and in inducing sweating.

Wormwood

Wormwood Native to temperate regions of Europe and northern Africa, wormwood—Artemisia absinthium L.—is recognized for its role in the production of the alcoholic beverage absinthe. Its bioactive profile includes dimeric guaianolides (absinthins) and monoterpene hydrocarbons (chamazulene). Wormwood is used to alleviate upset stomachs, loss of appetite, gall bladder and liver dysfunction, intestinal spasms, fever, worm infections, to enhance sexual desire, and induce sweating.

Valerian

Valerian Scientifically termed Valeriana officinalis, valerian, historically used as a perfume, is renowned for its medicinal properties. Widely employed in treating headaches, depression, insomnia, anxiety, premenstrual syndrome (PMS), and menopause-related abnormalities, valerian contains bioactive components like non-glycosidic iridoid esters, alkaloids, valepotriates, and flavonoids.

Turmeric

Turmeric Known as Indian saffron and with a medicinal history spanning almost 4000 years, turmeric, scientifically termed Curcuma longa, is a rhizomatous, herbaceous perennial. It contains various bioactive components, notably curcumin, curcumin II (demethoxycurcumin, 1-(4-hydroxy-3-methoxyphenyl)-7-(4-hydroxy-phenyl)-1,6-hepta-diene-3,5-dione), and curcumin III (bisdemethoxycurcumin, 1,7-bis(4-hydroxyphenyl)-1,6-heptadiene-3,5-dione).

Traditionally used in diverse medicinal practices for relieving gas, expelling worms, regulating menstruation, improving digestion, and managing arthritis, modern medicine has recognized its bioactive principles as potent antioxidants, anti-inflammatory, anti-mutagenic, antimicrobial, and anticancer agents.

Tulsi

Tulsi (Holy Basil) Referred to as "the queen of herbs" in Indian culture, Tulsi or holy basil has a rich history in Ayurvedic treatments for stress reduction, natural cleansing, and overall health enhancement. Its major bioactive components include ursolic acid, eugenol, rosmarinic acid, linalool, carvacrol, β caryophyllene, and oleanolic acid. Tulsi exhibits a diverse range of actions such as antimicrobial, anti-diabetic, adaptogenic, hepatoprotective, anti-carcinogenic, anti-inflammatory, radioprotective, neuroprotective, immunomodulatory, and cardioprotective effects.

Thyme

Thyme a fragrant perennial herb, Thyme (Thymus vulgaris) finds use in culinary, therapeutic, and decorative domains. Its bioactive profile encompasses carvacrol, thymol, ρ-cimeno, monoterpene hydrocarbons, γ-terpinen, γ-Tocopherol, and α-tocotrienol. Thyme is applied in treating acne, coughs, blood pressure irregularities, and may aid in boosting immunity, uplifting moods, and repelling pests.

Saffron

Saffron derived from the dried stigmas of Crocus sativus L., saffron grows mainly in mild and dry climates. With an ancient history of medicinal consumption, saffron is not only used as a food additive and colorant but also linked to therapeutic properties. Its phytochemicals—picrocrocin, safranal, and the carotenoid pigment crocin—give it distinct flavors, aromas, and a deep golden-yellow hue. Multiple studies have highlighted the therapeutic potential of these bioactive components in saffron.

Sage

Sage, scientifically termed Salvia officinalis, originates from the Mediterranean and is widely used as a flavor enhancer in various dishes, particularly in pork and poultry stuffings and

179

sausages. It can be utilized either fresh or dried. Sage contains numerous bioactive components like borneol, camphor, caryophyllene, cineole, elemene, humulene, ledene, pinene, thujone, rosmarinic acid, luteolin-7-glucoside, caffeic acid, 3-caffeoylquinic acid, chlorogenic acid, ellagic acid, epicatechin, epigallocatechin gallate, quercetin, rutin, and luteolin-7-glucoside.

Savory

Savory An annual herb native to North Africa and Eurasia, savory thrives abundantly, notably in France and Spain. Its extracts and essential oils contain coumarin, phenolic acids, hydroxybenzoic acids, flavonoids, linoleic acid, oleic acid, phytosterols (β-sitosterol and stigmasterol), and pectic polysaccharides, attributing to its antimicrobial, pesticidal, anti-parasitic, antioxidant, anti-inflammatory, hepatoprotective, analgesic, and anticancer properties. Recent studies have suggested its potential in treating cisplatin-induced liver injury in rats, showcasing effects akin to silymarin, a recognized hepatoprotective drug. Beyond its medicinal profile, savory's dried leaves, greenish-brown and aromatic, impart a mildly warm and sharp flavor to meals, especially in chicken dishes and stuffings.

Rosemary

Rosemary hailing from the Mediterranean, the fragrant herb rosemary, scientifically termed Salvia rosmarinus, finds use in culinary seasoning, perfumes, and possibly for health purposes. Its bioactive components include caffeic acid, carnosic acid, chlorogenic acid, monomeric acid, oleanolic acid, rosmarinic acid, ursolic acid, alpha-pinene, camphor, carnosol, eucalyptol, rosmadial, rosmanol, rosmaquinones A and B, secohinokio, and derivatives of eugenol and luteolin. Rosemary is used to alleviate muscle pain, enhance memory, support the circulatory and immune systems, and stimulate hair growth.

Parsley

Scientifically identified as Petroselinum crispum, parsley is a ubiquitous ingredient in food and beverages, serving as a garnish, condiment, and flavor enhancer. Parsley seed oil finds use in soap, cosmetic, and fragrance production. Its bioactive components include furanocoumarins (e.g., xanthoxin, trioxalen, and angelicin), essential oils (e.g., sesquiterpene hydrocarbons, monoterpene hydrocarbons and alcohols, furanocoumarins, aldehydes, and aromatic compounds), flavonoids (e.g., quercetin, apiol, myristicin, apigenin, luteolin, and their glycosides), carotenoids (e.g., neoxanthin, β-carotene, lutein, and violaxanthin), vitamins (e.g., tocopherols and A, C and B complexes), minerals (e.g., iron, zinc, calcium, and phosphorous), and fatty acids (e.g., linolenic and palmitic acid). It acts as a diuretic, reduces bloating, regulates blood pressure, and its rich vitamin K content stimulates bone growth and increases bone mineral density.

Oregano

Oregano, although associated with Italian and Spanish cuisine, actually originates from Northern Europe where it grows in the wild. Scientifically known as Origanum vulgare, this herb is used to address various conditions such as asthma, coughs, diarrhea, stomach aches, sores, muscle aches, and menstrual inflammatory disorders. Among its bioactive components are carvacrol, β-fenchyl alcohol, thymol, γ-terpinene, phenolic compounds, flavonoids, tocopherols, benzoic acid, rosmarinic acid, and cinnamic acid derivatives.

Nasturtium

Nasturtium scientifically termed Tropaeolum majus, nasturtiums, known for their peppery flavor, are often grown for ornamental purposes but can also serve as herbs. Their bioactive components include flavonoids, glucosinolates, anthocyanin, and fatty acids, contributing to potent antiseptic properties used for treating wounds and fungal infections. The pungent vapors are utilized to address bronchitis and other lung infections.

Mint

Mint, identified as Mentha piperita L., is a perennial herb boasting small, fragrant, serrated leaves in purple, pink, or white hues. Its bioactive components, encompassing eriocitrin, rosmarinic acid, luteolin 7-O-rutinoside, hesperidin, caffeic acid, ferulic acid, eugenol, pebrellin, gardenin B, and apigenin, are responsible for its various medicinal properties.

Milk Thistle

Milk Thistle scientifically known as Silybum marianum, milk thistle is revered for supporting liver functions and treating conditions like hepatitis, cirrhosis, jaundice, diabetes, and indigestion. Among its bioactive components are apigenin, silybonol, betaine, free fatty acids, silybin, silychristin, and silidianin.

Laurel

Laurel, scientifically termed Laurus nobilis, hails from the Mediterranean and is utilized for seasoning in various cuisines. Its bioactive components, including cinnamtannin B-1, trimeric A-type procyanidin, polyphenolic compounds, alkaloids, norisoprenoids, sugars, polysaccharides, organic acids, and tocopherols, contribute to its diverse applications, treating rheumatism, cardiac diseases, coughs, viral infections, diarrhea, and enhancing gastric secretion.

Lemon Grass

Lemon Grass Cymbopogon citratus, commonly known as lemon grass, belongs to a group of tropical herbs with a lemon-like flavor, growing in grassy clumps. Its bioactive components like myrcene, limonene, citral, geraniol, citronellol, geranyl acetate, neral, and nerol offer various health benefits such as reducing pain, fever, blood sugar, cholesterol, enhancing menstrual flow, and acting as an antioxidant.

Hyssop

Hyssop (Hyssopus officinalis) is a drought-resistant herb with bioactive components like diosmin, isopinocamphone, and pinocamphone, addressing nervous, pulmonary, uterine, digestive, and urinary system dysfunctions.

Gingko

Gingko Scientifically identified as Ginkgo biloba, gingko, an ancient tree species, utilizes its dried leaves for therapeutic purposes. Its bioactive components, including terpenoids, flavonoids, biflavonoids, organic acids, polyprenols, ginkgolides, and bilobalide, are utilized in treating memory issues and blood disorders.

Ginger

Ginger Zingiber officinale, known as ginger, is a perennial rhizome used in Indian and Asian cuisines. Its bioactive components—gingerols, shogaols, and paradols—offer various health benefits, including addressing motion sickness, indigestion, upset stomach, nausea, flu, and reducing blood insulin levels.

Garlic

Garlic scientifically termed Allium sativum, garlic is a widely used herb in cooking and medicinal practices. Bioactive components like diallyl thiosulfonate (allicin), diallyl sulfide, diallyl disulfide, diallyl trisulfide, E/Z-ajoene, S-allyl-cysteine, and S-allyl-cysteine sulfoxide (L-alliin) contribute to its benefits, such as reducing cancer risks, osteoarthritis, cardiovascular diseases, regulating blood cholesterol and pressure.

Fennel

Foeniculum vulgare, commonly known as fennel, is a tall

herb resembling dill, prized for its stems, leaves, and seeds. Its bioactive components encompass quinic acid, 4-O-caffeoylquinic acid, p-coumaric acid, rosmarinic acid, and chlorogenic acids, while its high vitamin C content supports immune health, collagen synthesis, tissue repair, cellular protection, blood sugar regulation, bone development, and wound healing.

Functional Properties of the Nutraceuticals

A multitude of plant-based bioactive compounds have displayed functional properties that suggest their potential in preventing various chronic ailments. It's widely recognized that fruits, vegetables, and medicinal herbs harbor diverse biological activities and offer antioxidant advantages. Phenolic compounds found in plant materials are directly associated with their antioxidant effects by impeding the generation of reactive oxygen species. This spotlight on nutraceuticals stems from their dual capacity in nutrition and therapeutic potential, garnering considerable attention. Herbal nutraceuticals play a crucial role in supporting and maintaining overall health, enhancing longevity, and elevating life quality. Research indicates the efficacy of nutraceuticals in addressing several conditions, including cancer, neurological issues, and cardiovascular ailments.

Diabetes

Diabetes, a metabolic disorder, emerges when the body inadequately produces or utilizes insulin. It affects roughly 422 million people worldwide and leads to approximately 1.5 million deaths yearly. The WHO highlighted critical issues in insulin and diabetes care globally, citing high prices, limited human insulin supply, market dominance by a few manufacturers, and deficient health systems as major barriers to access. Research indicates that plant-based diets, rich in minerals, vitamins, and phytochemicals, often possess anti-diabetic properties. Genistein, found in soybean seeds, exhibited promise in managing diabetes, enhancing insulin secretion in cell studies and improving insulin sensitivity in human trials. Grape seed proanthocyanidin extracts and those from Fagopyrum dibotrys demonstrated significant blood glucose-lowering effects in diabetic animals. Salvia officinalis extract, used in some regions, exhibited anti-diabetic potential by activating the peroxisome proliferator-activated receptor (PPAR).

Obesity

Obesity, characterized by excessive fat accumulation, is a widespread health concern. Plants, extracts, and compounds from plants are under investigation for their potential against obesity and associated conditions like non-alcoholic fatty liver disease (NAFLD). Lamiaceae plants are considered potential sources of nutraceuticals and phytochemicals for treating obesity and NAFLD. Amla consumption reduced liver lipid levels and oxidative stress, while Salvia officinalis leaf extract significantly inhibited pancreatic lipase, reducing body weight and obesity. Capsaicin, by activating TRPV1 channels, potentially promotes fat browning and reduces risks of hepatic steatosis and insulin resistance. Green tea extract AR25 showed promise in inhibiting lipases and promoting thermogenesis, suggesting suitability for obesity treatment.

Immunomodulation

Nutraceuticals derived from plants possess immunomo-dulatory properties. Compounds like rosmanol from sage and rosemary extracts exhibit anti-inflammatory effects by blocking certain pathways. Curcumin, oregano extracts, and their constituents have shown anti-inflammatory actions by regulating inflammatory factors and cytokines.

Dementia

The rising prevalence of dementia has led to increased usage of over-the-counter medications and nutraceuticals for cognitive issues. Terpenoids from Salvia lavandulaefolia demonstrate inhibitory activity against acetylcholinesterase, while sage shows positive effects on memory. Huperzine A from Huperzia serrata and caffeine from coffee exhibit neuroprotective properties, while lesser periwinkle and its derivative vinpocetine demonstrate potential cognitive benefits and improved blood flow to the brain in clinical trials.

Hypertension

Hypertension is a global health concern, but certain dietary components show promise in mitigating its effects. Hibiscus sabdariffa, known as sour tea, contains essential compounds that significantly lower blood pressure, as observed in pre-clinical animal studies. Ginger supplementation positively affects endothelial function and blood pressure. Saffron exhibits antioxidant properties, preventing blood pressure increases and aortic remodeling in hypertensive rats. Cinnamon, with its polyphenols, contributes to lowering blood pressure and glucose levels in animal models, potentially enhancing insulin sensitivity.

Antimicrobial Activity

Various plant-derived compounds possess potent antimicrobial effects. Samanea saman pod's tannins and phytochemicals show promise as natural antimicrobials. Larch bark extract demonstrates strong antibacterial activity against respiratory pathogens, suggesting its potential in nutraceutical formulations. Quercetin, found in vegetables and fruits, exhibits antiviral properties, including interference with SARS-CoV-2 replication in computer modeling. Psidium guajava displays significant antibacterial activity and is a candidate for effective antimicrobial agents. Thymus vulgaris essential oil shows potent bactericidal and antifungal activity, making it suitable for nutraceutical formulations or as a synergistic agent with antibiotics.

Apigenin from parsley exhibits anti-inflammatory properties by inhibiting enzymes and cytokines involved in inflammation.

Hypercholesterolemia

Red yeast rice, containing active compounds, significantly reduces total cholesterol concentrations. Berberine, found in medicinal plants like Coptis chinensis, lowers plasma lipids by regulating hepatic cholesterol and triglycerides. Meta-analyses show that soy protein intake reduces triglycerides, total cholesterol, and LDL cholesterol levels. Eleutherine americana Merr., or tiwai, may lower total cholesterol in individuals with hypercholesterolemia. Additionally, tree nuts have a beneficial impact on blood lipids, reducing triglycerides, LDL cholesterol, and total cholesterol levels, with the dose being the key factor in their effectiveness.

Safety, Quality and Regulatory Aspects of Herbal Nutraceuticals

The global usage of herbal medicine and dietary supplements is growing, employed either as medications or additives to boost overall well-being. Unlike conventional drugs, these supplements are categorized as food supplements by the FDA, subjected to different regulations. The FDA doesn't rigorously approve these supplements, only intervening when they're adulterated or misbranded. Concerningly, many supplements, including popular ones like echinacea, garlic, ginkgo, and St. John's wort, can have adverse effects, particularly when interacting with prescribed drugs.

These supplements are often available in crude extracts or commercial forms made from various plant parts, leading to variability in constituents and concentrations. This variance poses risks, including contaminants like heavy metals and banned ingredients. Regulatory bodies like DSHEA aim to balance the benefits and risks of these supplements, yet cases of liver injury or failure tied to certain products, such as

OxyElite Pro, have led to FDA warnings.

In the EU, herbal supplements are regulated under strict directives, requiring extensive usage history to be registered. However, online accessibility complicates proper identification and regulation of manufacturers, raising concerns about product quality and safety.

Educating consumers about the risks associated with herbal and dietary supplements is crucial. They should understand that not all supplements are risk-free, doses matter, and consulting healthcare professionals, especially when on other medications, is essential. If adverse effects occur, immediate cessation is recommended. It's advised to purchase supplements from reputable sources, although price isn't always indicative of quality. Special caution is urged for pregnant or nursing individuals, children, and those under medical care, as these groups are often advised against supplement use.

Conclusions

Nutraceuticals, derived from plants, offer health benefits and have seen a surge in the global market, including in India, driven by perceived therapeutic effects and increased interest in fitness and body toning. This review delves into the medicinal properties of these plant-based nutraceuticals, sourced from various herbs like aloe vera, anise, bay, caraway, dill, holy basil, thyme, saffron, sage, among others. These herbs contain vital bioactive components crucial for their functional potential, whose bioactivity heavily relies on effective extraction techniques.

Different extraction methods, from traditional ones like Soxhlet extraction to modern approaches such as supercritical fluid and microwave-assisted extraction, play a key role in obtaining high-quality bioactive compounds swiftly. Selecting the right extraction technique and subsequent purification processes ensure safeguarding the

potential components efficiently. The global nutraceutical market is projected to surpass USD 561 billion soon, with India contributing just 2%, indicating a need for increased production to meet the escalating demand.
Herbal nutraceuticals play a significant role in enhancing and sustaining quality of life by addressing widespread human diseases like cancer, diabetes, obesity, and hypertension. However, awareness about both the positive and adverse effects of these formulations is crucial. Future research should focus on understanding the therapeutic actions of bioactive compounds from herbs and developing strategies to identify and mitigate any adverse effects linked to herbal nutraceuticals.

References

1. Ivanišová, E.; Kačániová, M.; Savitskaya, T.D.A.; Grinshpan, D. Medicinal Herbs: Important Source of Bioactive Compounds for Food Industry. In *Herbs and Spices—New Processing Technologies*; IntechOpen: London, UK, 2021. [**Google Scholar**]
2. Priya, S.; Satheeshkumar, P.K. Natural Products from Plants. In *Functional and Preservative Properties of Phytochemicals*; Elsevier: Amsterdam, The Netherlands, 2020; pp. 145–163. [**Google Scholar**]
3. Majumder, R.; Das, C.K.; Mandal, M. Lead Bioactive Compounds of Aloe Vera as Potential Anticancer Agent. *Pharmacol. Res.* **2019**, *148*, 104416. [**Google Scholar**] [**CrossRef**]
4. Simpson, M. *Plant Systematics*, 3rd ed.; Academic Press: Cambridge, MA, USA, 2019; ISBN 9780128126288. [**Google Scholar**]
5. Añibarro-Ortega, M.; Pinela, J.; Barros, L.; Ćirić, A.; Silva, S.P.; Coelho, E.; Mocan, A.; Calhelha, R.C.; Soković, M.; Coimbra, M.A.; et al. Compositional

Features and Bioactive Properties of Aloe Vera Leaf (Fillet, Mucilage, and Rind) and Flower. *Antioxidants* **2019**, *8*, 444. [**Google Scholar**] [**CrossRef**] [**PubMed**][**Green Version**]

6. Özenver, N.; Saeed, M.; Demirezer, L.Ö.; Efferth, T. Aloe-Emodin as Drug Candidate for Cancer Therapy. *Oncotarget* **2018**, *9*, 17770–17796. [**Google Scholar**] [**CrossRef**] [**PubMed**][**Green Version**]

7. Huseini, H.; Kianbakht, S.; Hajiaghaee, R.; Dabaghian, F. Anti-Hyperglycemic and Anti-Hypercholesterolemic Effects of Aloe Vera Leaf Gel in Hyperlipidemic Type 2 Diabetic Patients: A Randomized Double-Blind Placebo-Controlled Clinical Trial. *Planta Med.* **2012**, *78*, 311–316. [**Google Scholar**] [**CrossRef**] [**PubMed**][**Green Version**]

8. Zhao, C.; Jia, Y.; Lu, F. Angelica Stem: A Potential Low-Cost Source of Bioactive Phthalides and Phytosterols. *Molecules* **2018**, *23*, 3065. [**Google Scholar**] [**CrossRef**][**Green Version**]

9. Bettaieb Rebey, I.; Aidi Wannes, W.; Ben Kaab, S.; Bourgou, S.; Tounsi, M.S.; Ksouri, R.; Fauconnier, M.L. Bioactive Compounds and Antioxidant Activity of Pimpinella Anisum L. Accessions at Different Ripening Stages. *Sci. Hortic.* **2019**, *246*, 453–461. [**Google Scholar**] [**CrossRef**]

10. Sun, W.; Shahrajabian, M.H.; Cheng, Q. Anise (*Pimpinella Anisum* L.), a Dominant Spice and Traditional Medicinal Herb for Both Food and Medicinal Purposes. *Cogent Biol.* **2019**, *5*, 1673688. [**Google Scholar**] [**CrossRef**]

11. Ju, B.; Chen, B.; Zhang, X.; Han, C.; Jiang, A. Purification and Characterization of Bioactive Compounds from Styela Clava. *J. Chem.* **2014**, *2014*, 525141. [**Google Scholar**] [**CrossRef**][**Green Version**]

12. Sun, C.; Huang, H.; Xu, C.; Li, X.; Chen, K. Biological Activities of Extracts from Chinese Bayberry (Myrica Rubra Sieb. et Zucc.): A Review. *Plant Foods Hum. Nutr.* **2013**, *68*, 97–106. [**Google Scholar**] [**CrossRef**]

13. Zhang, X.; Huang, H.; Zhang, Q.; Fan, F.; Xu, C.; Sun, C.; Li, X.; Chen, K. Phytochemical Characterization of Chinese Bayberry (Myrica Rubra Sieb. et Zucc.) of 17 Cultivars and Their Antioxidant Properties. *Int. J. Mol. Sci.* **2015**, *16*, 12467–12481. [**Google Scholar**] [**CrossRef**][**Green Version**]

14. Pelc, M.; Przybyszewska, E.; Przybył, J.L.; Capecka, E.; Bączek, K.; Węglarz, Z. Chemical variability of great burnet (*Sanguisorba officinalis* L.) growing wild in poland. *Acta Hortic.* **2011**, *925*, 97–101. [**Google Scholar**] [**CrossRef**]

15. Debbabi, H.; El Mokni, R.; Chaieb, I.; Nardoni, S.; Maggi, F.; Caprioli, G.; Hammami, S. Chemical Composition, Antifungal and Insecticidal Activities of the Essential Oils from Tunisian Clinopodium Nepeta Subsp. Nepeta and Clinopodium Nepeta Subsp. Glandulosum. *Molecules* **2020**, *25*, 2137. [**Google Scholar**] [**CrossRef**]

16. Johri, R. Cuminum Cyminum and Carum Carvi: An Update. *Pharmacogn. Rev.* **2011**, *5*, 63. [**Google Scholar**] [**CrossRef**] [**PubMed**][**Green Version**]

17. Degner, S.C.; Papoutsis, A.J.; Romagnolo, D.F. Health Benefits of Traditional Culinary and Medicinal Mediterranean Plants. In *Complementary and Alternative Therapies and the Aging Population*; Elsevier: Amsterdam, The Netherlands, 2009; pp. 541–562. [**Google Scholar**]

18. Nour, V.; Trandafir, I.; Cosmulescu, S. Bioactive Compounds, Antioxidant Activity and Nutritional Quality of Different Culinary Aromatic Herbs. *Not. Bot.*

Horti Agrobot. Cluj-Napoca **2017**, *45*, 179–184. [**Google Scholar**] [**CrossRef**][**Green Version**]

19. Hadisaputri, Y.E.; Miyazaki, T.; Suzuki, S.; Kubo, N.; Zuhrotun, A.; Yokobori, T.; Abdulah, R.; Yazawa, S.; Kuwano, H. Molecular Characterization of Antitumor Effects of the Rhizome Extract from Curcuma Zedoaria on Human Esophageal Carcinoma Cells. *Int. J. Oncol.* **2015**, *47*, 2255–2263. [**Google Scholar**] [**CrossRef**] [**PubMed**][**Green Version**]

20. Msaada, K.; Salem, N.; Bachrouch, O.; Bousselmi, S.; Tammar, S.; Alfaify, A.; Al Sane, K.; Ben Ammar, W.; Azeiz, S.; Haj Brahim, A.; et al. Chemical Composition and Antioxidant and Antimicrobial Activities of Wormwood (*Artemisia Absinthium* L.) Essential Oils and Phenolics. *J. Chem.* **2015**, *2015*, 804658. [**Google Scholar**] [**CrossRef**][**Green Version**]

21. Ma, Y.; Pei, S.; He, N.; Lai, Q.; Zhuang, M.; Bian, Z.; Lin, C. A Narrative Review of Botanical Characteristics, Phytochemistry and Pharmacology of Valeriana Jatamansi Jones. *Longhua Chinese Med.* **2021**, *4*, 5. [**Google Scholar**] [**CrossRef**]

22. Sharifi-Rad, J.; El Rayess, Y.; Rizk, A.A.; Sadaka, C.; Zgheib, R.; Zam, W.; Sestito, S.; Rapposelli, S.; Neffe-Skocińska, K.; Zielińska, D.; et al. Turmeric and Its Major Compound Curcumin on Health: Bioactive Effects and Safety Profiles for Food, Pharmaceutical, Biotechnological and Medicinal Applications. *Front. Pharmacol.* **2020**, *11*, 01021. [**Google Scholar**] [**CrossRef**]

23. Yamani, H.A.; Pang, E.C.; Mantri, N.; Deighton, M.A. Antimicrobial Activity of Tulsi (Ocimum Tenuiflorum) Essential Oil and Their Major Constituents against Three Species of Bacteria. *Front. Microbiol.* **2016**, *7*, 681. [**Google Scholar**] [**CrossRef**][**Green Version**]

24. Nieto, G. A Review on Applications and Uses of Thymus in the Food Industry. *Plants* **2020**, *9*, 961. [**Google Scholar**] [**CrossRef**]
25. Rahaiee, S.; Moini, S.; Hashemi, M.; Shojaosadati, S.A. Evaluation of Antioxidant Activities of Bioactive Compounds and Various Extracts Obtained from Saffron (*Crocus sativus* L.): A Review. *J. Food Sci. Technol.* **2015**, *52*, 1881–1888. [**Google Scholar**] [**CrossRef**] [**PubMed**][**Green Version**]
26. Ghorbani, A.; Esmaeilizadeh, M. Pharmacological Properties of Salvia Officinalis and Its Components. *J. Tradit. Complement. Med.* **2017**, *7*, 433–440. [**Google Scholar**] [**CrossRef**] [**PubMed**]
27. Clavel-Coibrié, E.; Sales, J.R.; da Silva, A.M.; Barroca, M.J.; Sousa, I.; Raymundo, A. Sarcocornia Perennis: A Salt Substitute in Savory Snacks. *Foods* **2021**, *10*, 3110. [**Google Scholar**] [**CrossRef**]
28. Fierascu, I.; Dinu-Pirvu, C.E.; Fierascu, R.C.; Velescu, B.S.; Anuta, V.; Ortan, A.; Jinga, V. Phytochemical Profile and Biological Activities of Satureja Hortensis L.: A Review of the Last Decade. *Molecules* **2018**, *23*, 2458. [**Google Scholar**] [**CrossRef**] [**PubMed**][**Green Version**]
29. de Oliveira, J.R.; Camargo, S.E.A.; de Oliveira, L.D. *Rosmarinus officinalis* L. (Rosemary) as Therapeutic and Prophylactic Agent. *J. Biomed. Sci.* **2019**, *26*, 5. [**Google Scholar**] [**CrossRef**] [**PubMed**]
30. Liberal, Â.; Fernandes, Â.; Polyzos, N.; Petropoulos, S.A.; Dias, M.I.; Pinela, J.; Petrović, J.; Soković, M.; Ferreira, I.C.F.R.; Barros, L. Bioactive Properties and Phenolic Compound Profiles of Turnip-Rooted, Plain-Leafed and Curly-Leafed Parsley Cultivars. *Molecules* **2020**, *25*, 5606. [**Google Scholar**] [**CrossRef**]

31. Atar, H.; Çölgeçen, H. Bioactive Compounds of Oregano Seeds. In *Nuts and Seeds in Health and Disease Prevention*; Elsevier: Amsterdam, The Netherlands, 2020; pp. 73–77. [Google Scholar]
32. Klimek-Szczykutowicz, M.; Dziurka, M.; Blažević, I.; Đulović, A.; Granica, S.; Korona-Glowniak, I.; Ekiert, H.; Szopa, A. Phytochemical and Biological Activity Studies on *Nasturtium officinale* (Watercress) Microshoot Cultures Grown in RITA® Temporary Immersion Systems. *Molecules* 2020, *25*, 5257. [Google Scholar] [CrossRef]
33. Brown, N.; John, J.A.; Shahidi, F. Polyphenol Composition and Antioxidant Potential of Mint Leaves. *Food Prod. Process. Nutr.* 2019, *1*, 1. [Google Scholar] [CrossRef][Green Version]
34. Aziz, M.; Saeed, F.; Ahmad, N.; Ahmad, A.; Afzaal, M.; Hussain, S.; Mohamed, A.A.; Alamri, M.S.; Anjum, F.M. Biochemical Profile of Milk Thistle (*Silybum Marianum* L.) with Special Reference to Silymarin Content. *Food Sci. Nutr.* 2021, *9*, 244–250. [Google Scholar] [CrossRef]
35. Rubió, L.; Motilva, M.-J.; Romero, M.-P. Recent Advances in Biologically Active Compounds in Herbs and Spices: A Review of the Most Effective Antioxidant and Anti-Inflammatory Active Principles. *Crit. Rev. Food Sci. Nutr.* 2013, *53*, 943–953. [Google Scholar] [CrossRef]
36. Nasri, H.; Baradaran, A.; Shirzad, H.; Rafieian-Kopaei, M. New Concepts in Nutraceuticals as Alternative for Pharmaceuticals. *Int. J. Prev. Med.* 2014, *5*, 1487–1499. [Google Scholar] [PubMed]
37. Ohno, T.; Kato, N.; Ishii, C.; Shimizu, M.; Ito, Y.; Tomono, S.; Kawazu, S. Genistein Augments Cyclic Adenosine 3'5'-Monophosphate (CAMP) Accumulation and Insulin Release in Min6 Cells. *Endocr.*

Res. **1993**, *19*, 273–285. [Google Scholar] [CrossRef] [PubMed]
38. Villa, P.; Costantini, B.; Suriano, R.; Perri, C.; Macrì, F.; Ricciardi, L.; Panunzi, S.; Lanzone, A. The Differential Effect of the Phytoestrogen Genistein on Cardiovascular Risk Factors in Postmenopausal Women: Relationship with the Metabolic Status. *J. Clin. Endocrinol. Metab.* **2009**, *94*, 552–558. [Google Scholar] [CrossRef] [PubMed][Green Version]
39. Wang, Y.; Zhang, G.; Xu, B.; Yao, D.; Zhang, D. Effect of Grape Seed Proanthocyanidin Extracts on Blood Glucose of Diabetic Mice. *Nat. Prod. Res. Dev.* **2012**, *23*, 1191. [Google Scholar]
40. Li, X.; Liu, J.; Chang, Q.; Zhou, Z.; Han, R.; Liang, Z. Antioxidant and Antidiabetic Activity of Proanthocyanidins from Fagopyrum Dibotrys. *Molecules* **2021**, *26*, 2417. [Google Scholar] [CrossRef] [PubMed]
41. Christensen, K.B.; Jørgensen, M.; Kotowska, D.; Petersen, R.K.; Kristiansen, K.; Christensen, L.P. Activation of the Nuclear Receptor PPARγ by Metabolites Isolated from Sage (*Salvia officinalis* L.). *J. Ethnopharmacol.* **2010**, *132*, 127–133. [Google Scholar] [CrossRef]
42. Diab, F.; Zbeeb, H.; Baldini, F.; Portincasa, P.; Khalil, M.; Vergani, L. The Potential of Lamiaceae Herbs for Mitigation of Overweight, Obesity, and Fatty Liver: Studies and Perspectives. *Molecules* **2022**, *27*, 5043. [Google Scholar] [CrossRef]
43. Nijhawan, P.; Behl, T. Nutraceuticals in the Management of Obesity. *Obes. Med.* **2020**, *17*, 100168. [Google Scholar] [CrossRef]
44. Ninomiya, K.; Matsuda, H.; Shimoda, H.; Nishida, N.; Kasajima, N.; Yoshino, T.; Morikawa, T.; Yoshikawa, M. Carnosic Acid, a New Class of Lipid Absorption

Inhibitor from Sage. *Bioorg. Med. Chem. Lett.* **2004**, *14*, 1943–1946. [**Google Scholar**] [**CrossRef**]

45. Baskaran, P.; Krishnan, V.; Ren, J.; Thyagarajan, B. Capsaicin Induces Browning of White Adipose Tissue and Counters Obesity by Activating TRPV1 Channel-Dependent Mechanisms. *Br. J. Pharmacol.* **2016**, *173*, 2369–2389. [**Google Scholar**] [**CrossRef**][**Green Version**]

46. Kang, J.-H.; Tsuyoshi, G.; Han, I.-S.; Kawada, T.; Kim, Y.M.; Yu, R. Dietary Capsaicin Reduces Obesity-Induced Insulin Resistance and Hepatic Steatosis in Obese Mice Fed a High-Fat Diet. *Obesity* **2010**, *18*, 780–787. [**Google Scholar**] [**CrossRef**] [**PubMed**]

47. Chantre, P.; Lairon, D. Recent Findings of Green Tea Extract AR25 (Exolise) and Its Activity for the Treatment of Obesity. *Phytomedicine* **2002**, *9*, 3–8. [**Google Scholar**] [**CrossRef**] [**PubMed**]

48. Lai, C.-S.; Lee, J.H.; Ho, C.-T.; Bin Liu, C.; Wang, J.-M.; Wang, Y.-J.; Pan, M.-H. Rosmanol Potently Inhibits Lipopolysaccharide-Induced INOS and COX-2 Expression through Downregulating MAPK, NF-KB, STAT3 and C/EBP Signaling Pathways. *J. Agric. Food Chem.* **2009**, *57*, 10990–10998. [**Google Scholar**] [**CrossRef**] [**PubMed**]

49. Aggarwal, B.B.; Sung, B. Pharmacological Basis for the Role of Curcumin in Chronic Diseases: An Age-Old Spice with Modern Targets. *Trends Pharmacol. Sci.* **2009**, *30*, 85–94. [**Google Scholar**] [**CrossRef**]

50. Ocaña-Fuentes, A.; Arranz-Gutiérrez, E.; Señorans, F.J.; Reglero, G. Supercritical Fluid Extraction of Oregano (*Origanum vulgare*) Essentials Oils: Anti-Inflammatory Properties Based on Cytokine Response on THP-1 Macrophages. *Food Chem. Toxicol.* **2010**, *48*, 1568–1575. [**Google Scholar**] [**CrossRef**]

51. Savelev, S.; Okello, E.; Perry, N.S.L.; Wilkins, R.M.; Perry, E.K. Synergistic and Antagonistic Interactions of Anticholinesterase Terpenoids in Salvia Lavandulaefolia Essential Oil. *Pharmacol. Biochem. Behav.* **2003**, *75*, 661–668. [**Google Scholar**] [**CrossRef**]

52. Akhondzadeh, S.; Noroozian, M.; Mohammadi, M.; Ohadinia, S.; Jamshidi, A.H.; Khani, M. Salvia Officinalis Extract in the Treatment of Patients with Mild to Moderate Alzheimer's Disease: A Double Blind, Randomized and Placebo-Controlled Trial. *J. Clin. Pharm. Ther.* **2003**, *28*, 53–59. [**Google Scholar**] [**CrossRef**]

53. Howes, M.-J.R.; Houghton, P.J. Traditional Medicine for Memory Enhancement. In *Herbal Drugs: Ethnomedicine to Modern Medicine*; Springer: Berlin/Heidelberg, Germany, 2009; pp. 239–291. [**Google Scholar**]

54. Eskelinen, M.H.; Ngandu, T.; Tuomilehto, J.; Soininen, H.; Kivipelto, M. Midlife Coffee and Tea Drinking and the Risk of Late-Life Dementia: A Population-Based CAIDE Study. *J. Alzheimer's Dis.* **2009**, *16*, 85–91. [**Google Scholar**] [**CrossRef**][**Green Version**]

55. Nyakas, C.; Felszeghy, K.; Szabó, R.; Keijser, J.N.; Luiten, P.G.M.; Szombathelyi, Z.; Tihanyi, K. Neuroprotective Effects of Vinpocetine and Its Major Metabolite Cis -Apovincaminic Acid on NMDA-Induced Neurotoxicity in a Rat Entorhinal Cortex Lesion Model. *CNS Neurosci. Ther.* **2009**, *15*, 89–99. [**Google Scholar**] [**CrossRef**]

56. Inuwa, I.; Ali, B.H.; Al-Lawati, I.; Beegam, S.; Ziada, A.; Blunden, G. Long-Term Ingestion of Hibiscus Sabdariffa Calyx Extract Enhances Myocardial Capillarization in the Spontaneously Hypertensive Rat. *Exp. Biol. Med.* **2012**, *237*, 563–569. [**Google Scholar**] [**CrossRef**]

57. Azimi, P.; Ghiasvand, R.; Feizi, A.; Hosseinzadeh, J.; Bahreynian, M.; Hariri, M.; Khosravi-Boroujeni, H. Effect of Cinnamon, Cardamom, Saffron and Ginger Consumption on Blood Pressure and a Marker of Endothelial Function in Patients with Type 2 Diabetes Mellitus: A Randomized Controlled Clinical Trial. *Blood Press.* **2016**, *25*, 133–140. [**Google Scholar**] [**CrossRef**] [**PubMed**]

58. Alizadeh, R.N.; Fatemeh Roozbeh Saravi, M.; Pourumir, M.; Jalali, F.; Moghadamnia, A.A. Investigation of the Effect of Ginger on the Lipid Levels. A Double Blind Controlled Clinical Trial. *Saudi Med. J.* **2008**, *29*, 1280–1284. [**Google Scholar**]

59. Shelly, T.E.; McInnis, D.O.; Pahio, E.; Edu, J. Aromatherapy in the Mediterranean Fruit Fly (Diptera: Tephritidae): Sterile Males Exposed to Ginger Root Oil in Prerelease Storage Boxes Display Increased Mating Competitiveness in Field-Cage Trials. *J. Econ. Entomol.* **2004**, *97*, 846–853. [**Google Scholar**] [**CrossRef**] [**PubMed**]

60. Su, X.; Yuan, C.; Wang, L.; Chen, R.; Li, X.; Zhang, Y.; Liu, C.; Liu, X.; Liang, W.; Xing, Y. The Beneficial Effects of Saffron Extract on Potential Oxidative Stress in Cardiovascular Diseases. *Oxid. Med. Cell Longev.* **2021**, *2021*, 6699821. [**Google Scholar**] [**CrossRef**]

61. Nasiri, Z.; Sameni, H.R.; Vakili, A.; Jarrahi, M.; Khorasani, M.Z. Dietary Saffron Reduced the Blood Pressure and Prevented Remodeling of the Aorta in L-NAME-Induced Hypertensive Rats. *Iran. J. Basic Med. Sci.* **2015**, *18*, 1143–1146. [**Google Scholar**]

62. Preuss, H.G.; Echard, B.; Polansky, M.M.; Anderson, R. Whole Cinnamon and Aqueous Extracts Ameliorate Sucrose-Induced Blood Pressure Elevations in

Spontaneously Hypertensive Rats. *J. Am. Coll. Nutr.* **2006**, *25*, 144–150. [**Google Scholar**] [**CrossRef**]

63. Akilen, R.; Tsiami, A.; Devendra, D.; Robinson, N. Glycated Haemoglobin and Blood Pressure-Lowering Effect of Cinnamon in Multi-Ethnic Type 2 Diabetic Patients in the UK: A Randomized, Placebo-Controlled, Double-Blind Clinical Trial. *Diabet. Med.* **2010**, *27*, 1159–1167. [**Google Scholar**] [**CrossRef**]

64. Ukoha, P.O.; Cemaluk, E.A.C.; Nnamdi, O.L.; Madus, E.P. Tannins and Other Phytochemical of the Samanaea Saman Pods and Their Antimicrobial Activities. *Afr. J. Pure Appl. Chem.* **2011**, *5*, 237–244. [**Google Scholar**]

65. Faggian, M.; Bernabè, G.; Ferrari, S.; Francescato, S.; Baratto, G.; Castagliuolo, I.; Dall'Acqua, S.; Peron, G. Polyphenol-Rich Larix Decidua Bark Extract with Antimicrobial Activity against Respiratory-Tract Pathogens: A Novel Bioactive Ingredient with Potential Pharmaceutical and Nutraceutical Applications. *Antibiotics* **2021**, *10*, 789. [**Google Scholar**] [**CrossRef**]

66. Derosa, G.; Maffioli, P.; D'Angelo, A.; Di Pierro, F. A Role for Quercetin in Coronavirus Disease 2019 (COVID-19). *Phyther. Res.* **2021**, *35*, 1230–1236. [**Google Scholar**] [**CrossRef**]

67. Chanda, S.; Kaneria, M. Indian Nutraceutical Plant Leaves as a Potential Source of Natural Antimicrobial Agents. In *Science against Microbial Pathogens: Communicating Current Research and Technological Advances*; FORMATEX Research Center: Badajoz, Spain, 2011; pp. 1251–1259. [**Google Scholar**]

68. Al Maqtari, M.A.A.; Alghalibi, S.M.; Alhamzy, E.H. Chemical Composition and Antimicrobial Activity of Essential Oil of Thymus Vulgaris from Yemen. *Türk. Biyokim. Derg. Turkish J. Biochem.* **2011**, *36*, 342–349. [**Google Scholar**]

69. Salehi, B.; Venditti, A.; Sharifi-Rad, M.; Kręgiel, D.; Sharifi-Rad, J.; Durazzo, A.; Lucarini, M.; Santini, A.; Souto, E.; Novellino, E.; et al. The Therapeutic Potential of Apigenin. *Int. J. Mol. Sci.* **2019**, *20*, 1305. [**Google Scholar**] [**CrossRef**] [**PubMed**][**Green Version**]

70. Heber, D.; Yip, I.; Ashley, J.M.; Elashoff, D.A.; Elashoff, R.M.; Go, V.L.W. Cholesterol-Lowering Effects of a Proprietary Chinese Red-Yeast-Rice Dietary Supplement. *Am. J. Clin. Nutr.* **1999**, *69*, 231–236. [**Google Scholar**] [**CrossRef**] [**PubMed**][**Green Version**]

71. Brusq, J.-M.; Ancellin, N.; Grondin, P.; Guillard, R.; Martin, S.; Saintillan, Y.; Issandou, M. Inhibition of Lipid Synthesis through Activation of AMP Kinase: An Additional Mechanism for the Hypolipidemic Effects of Berberine. *J. Lipid Res.* **2006**, *47*, 1281–1288. [**Google Scholar**] [**CrossRef**] [**PubMed**][**Green Version**]

72. Anderson, J.W.; Johnstone, B.M.; Cook-Newell, M.E. Meta-Analysis of the Effects of Soy Protein Intake on Serum Lipids. *N. Engl. J. Med.* **1995**, *333*, 276–282. [**Google Scholar**] [**CrossRef**]

73. Saraheni, S.; David, W. Effect of Herbal Drink Plants Tiwai (Eleutherine Americana Merr) on Lipid Profile of Hypercholesterolemia Patients. *Int. Food Res. J.* **2014**, *21*, 1163–1167. [**Google Scholar**]

74. Del Gobbo, L.C.; Falk, M.C.; Feldman, R.; Lewis, K.; Mozaffarian, D. Effects of Tree Nuts on Blood Lipids, Apolipoproteins, and Blood Pressure: Systematic Review, Meta-Analysis, and Dose-Response of 61 Controlled Intervention Trials. *Am. J. Clin. Nutr.* **2015**, *102*, 1347–1356. [**Google Scholar**] [**CrossRef**][**Green Version**]

75. Thakkar, S.; Anklam, E.; Xu, A.; Ulberth, F.; Li, J.; Li, B.; Hugas, M.; Sarma, N.; Crerar, S.; Swift, S.; et al. Regulatory Landscape of Dietary Supplements and

Herbal Medicines from a Global Perspective. *Regul. Toxicol. Pharmacol.* **2020**, *114*, 104647. [**Google Scholar**] [**CrossRef**]
76. Williams, C.T. Herbal Supplements. *Nurs. Clin. N. Am.* **2021**, *56*, 1–21. [**Google Scholar**] [**CrossRef**]
77. Bunchorntavakul, C.; Reddy, K.R. Review Article: Herbal and Dietary Supplement Hepatotoxicity. *Aliment. Pharmacol. Ther.* **2013**, *37*, 3–17. [**Google Scholar**] [**CrossRef**]
78. De Boer, Y.S.; Sherker, A.H. Herbal and Dietary Supplement–Induced Liver Injury. *Clin. Liver Dis.* **2017**, *21*, 135–149. [**Google Scholar**] [**CrossRef**][**Green Version**]
79. Ko, R. Safety of Ethnic & Imported Herbal and Dietary Supplements. *Clin. Toxicol.* **2006**, *44*, 611–616. [**Google Scholar**] [**CrossRef**] [**PubMed**]

Chapter-14

Nutraceutical and Therapeutical Potential of See Weeds

Introduction

Seaweeds have been part of human diets for millennia, particularly in Asian countries like China, Japan, and South Korea. While their culinary use originated in these regions, the popularity of seaweed has spread to the Western world, finding its way into the USA, South America, and Europe due to its functional properties and introduction in various cuisines. Today, seaweed is highly regarded as a versatile food ingredient, utilized directly or indirectly in preparing diverse foods and beverages. Its significance extends beyond just food—it's employed in the food industry, as part of fertilizers, animal feed supplements, and additives for functional foods.

Nutritionally, seaweeds pack a punch: low in calories yet rich in vitamins, minerals, essential trace elements, poly-unsaturated fatty acids, proteins, polysaccharides, and dietary fibers. Beyond regular consumption, numerous studies highlight the health benefits of seaweed supplementation in conjunction with a balanced diet. For instance, it's been linked to reduced depressive symptoms in pregnant women in Japan and a decreased risk of suicide in adults. Regular consumption has also shown promise in lowering the risk of diabetes mellitus in the Korean population.

Moreover, seaweed isn't just about nutrition; its medicinal properties have been acknowledged historically. Seaweeds have been used to address iodine deficiency-related conditions like goitre. Research indicates that various types of seaweed possess therapeutic effects against non-communicable diseases such as inflammation, obesity, diabetes, hypertension, and even viral infections. Clinical studies have suggested that certain seaweed types might lower the risk of breast cancer or alleviate osteoarthritis symptoms.

Seaweeds are also recognized for their antioxidant capacities and bioactive polyphenolic compounds. Studies have hinted at their potential in HIV protection, largely attributed to specific compounds found in algae. Additionally, they've shown promise in preventing cancer and addressing metabolic syndrome related to obesity, cardiovascular diseases, diabetes, and chronic inflammation.

The dietary fibers found in seaweed, both fermentable and insoluble, are crucial for digestive health. They contribute to mitigating issues like colorectal cancer, gastrointestinal inflammation, and support probiotics and other adverse health conditions.

Although some evidence suggests that the impact of bioactive compounds from seaweed on the human body might be moderate and short-term, regular consumption as part of a daily diet could have significant long-term benefits. Hence, this review focuses on exploring the therapeutic role of seaweed-derived compounds as nutraceuticals or functional food ingredients for maintaining health and preventing diseases. It delves into the scientific understanding of primary and secondary metabolites, their functional properties, bioavailability, and their influence on body metabolism.

Bioactive compounds from seaweed

Polysaccharides derived from seaweed or microalgae exhibit a diverse array of beneficial properties, including anti-inflammatory, antioxidant, anticarcinogenic, anticoagulant, and antiviral activities. Sulfated polysaccharides found abundantly in seaweed contribute significantly to its bioactivity, capable of interacting with various cellular proteins and textures. Within seaweed, polysaccharides stand as the most crucial macromolecule, constituting over 80% of its weight.

Seaweed boasts a higher concentration of protein compared to terrestrial plant sources like soybeans or pulses. Notably, red seaweed leads in the ratio of essential to non-essential amino acids (EAA/NEAA) with a ratio of 0.98–1.02, followed by green seaweed at 0.72–0.97, and brown seaweed at 0.73.

Vitamins play a pivotal role in metabolic pathways and enzyme co-factor synthesis. Seaweeds emerge as an exceptional source of vitamins, encompassing both essential and non-essential types within their cellular structure. Certain seaweeds such as Porphyra umbilicalis, Himanthalia elongata, and Gracilaria changii exhibit notably high levels of Vitamin C compared to typical land vegetables.

In terms of phytochemicals, macroalgae harbor an extensive range of secondary metabolites that have captured the scientific community's interest for their potential bioactivity, surpassing even some plant sources. Brown algae, for instance, contain substantial amounts of phloroglucinol, serving as a nutraceutical agent with associated health benefits. Seaweeds demonstrate a spectrum of biological activities such as antioxidant, antiproliferative, anti-inflammatory, antidiabetic, anti-HIV, and even anti-Alzheimer's activity, as observed in vitro studies.

Therapeutic properties of seaweed-derived compounds

Nutraceuticals, beyond their nutritional value, serve as supplements or medicinal substances offering physiological benefits and protection against chronic diseases. Their rising popularity owes to the nutritional, safety, and therapeutic effects they provide. These supplements address nutrient deficiencies, aid in treating specific ailments, and even support overall health, aging, and longevity.

With the global population expanding and certain regions facing food crisis challenges, there's a push towards sustainable sources for nutraceutical production. Seaweeds, or Macro Algae, have gained attention for their ability to synthesize high-value molecules through photosynthesis, making them a reliable source of abundant nutritional compounds.

Serious global health concerns include cancer, diabetes, inflammation, and chronic cardiovascular diseases. While chemotherapy and synthetic drugs have been widely used, their side effects like toxicity, drug tolerance, and metabolic disorders drive the search for natural bioactive alternatives to prevent these diseases. Seaweeds stand out as one of the richest sources of biologically active metabolites, encompassing polysaccharides, unsaturated fatty acids, phenols, peptides, terpenoids, and other unique compounds. These components exhibit a spectrum of effects such as antioxidant, antiviral, anticoagulant, antibacterial, and antitumor properties. Brown, red, and green seaweeds contain various active substances with immense potential across agricultural, edible, and medical applications, as depicted in Figure 1 illustrating seaweed's therapeutic applications.

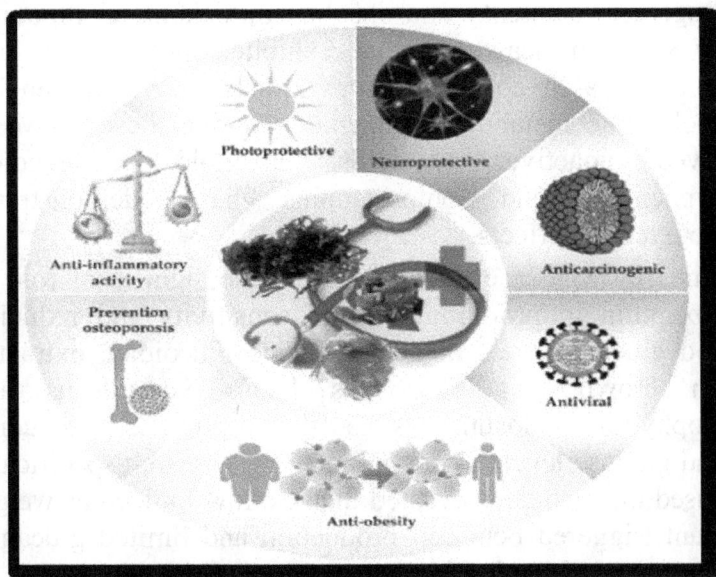

Figure 1 : Application of see weeds in different therapeutic purpose

Seaweeds, or algae, stand out as vital sources of novel therapeutic compounds with immense potential for human health. Bioactive substances extracted from seaweed play a pivotal role in preventing various diseases in humans. Within seaweeds, biomolecules like polysaccharides, pigments, fatty acids, polyphenols, and peptides have undergone rigorous testing, showcasing diverse and beneficial biological properties. These properties hold promising potential for the development of functional foods and nutraceuticals. Surprisingly, while green seaweeds, or Green Macro Algae, are rich reservoirs of bioactive compounds, they remain underutilized in the realms of nutraceuticals and pharmaceuticals, presenting an opportunity for further exploration and application.

Effect on glucose metabolism

In recent years, the landscape of diabetes treatment has seen the emergence of various new drugs, encompassing oral hypoglycemic agents and insulin mimickers. Compounds derived from seaweed have exhibited both safety and effectiveness in combating type-2-diabetes by influencing carbohydrate metabolism enzymes. Among these seaweed-derived bioactives, alkaloids, flavonoids, carotenoids, polyphenols, and phlorotannins have demonstrated hypoglycemic effects.

Studies by Maeda et al. highlighted the significant role of fucoxanthin in promoting insulin sensitivity and reducing blood glucose levels in diabetic mice. Fucoidan, extracted from brown algae such as Fucus vesiculosus and Ascophyllum nodosum, has also shown promise in reducing blood glucose levels in animal models. Research specifically focused on fucoidan revealed that the low molecular weight variant triggered beta cell production and limited glucagon secretion, resulting in blood glucose reversal.

Notably, fucoidan from Ascophyllum nodosum exhibited

more pronounced activity on α-amylose and α-glucosidase compared to its counterpart from Fucus vesiculosus. The efficacy of fucoidan in inhibiting α-glucosidase activity appeared to be species-specific and contingent upon the harvesting period. For instance, fucoidan extracted from A. nodosum during autumn exhibited significant α-glucosidase inhibition compared to other seasons. Similarly, varying levels of α-glucosidase inhibition were observed between fucoidan from A. nodosum and F. vesiculosus, with A. nodosum fucoidan displaying stronger inhibition.

The mechanism behind fucoidan's inhibitory action remains uncertain, but it may involve electrostatic interactions between sulfate groups and enzymes, as well as the viscosity of fucoidan impacting diffusivity in solvents. Additionally, the bioactivity of seaweed fucoidan is contingent upon its molecular weight, with low molecular weight fucoidan exhibiting higher absorption and bioavailability than high molecular weight variants.

Moreover, crude seaweed extracts, such as methanolic extracts of E. stolonifera, demonstrated potent inhibition of α-glucosidase and significantly reduced plasma glucose levels in diabetic mice. Analysis revealed that phlorotannin phenolic compounds within the extract were responsible for the hypoglycemic effect.

Interestingly, research suggests that polyphenolic compounds exhibit greater hypoglycemic potency compared to polysaccharide fractions of seaweeds. While the polyphenolic fraction of A. nodosum showed significant α-glucosidase inhibition at low concentrations, the polysaccharide fraction did not achieve the same level of reduction at similar concentrations.

Effect on cell proliferation

Evidence suggests that fucoidan, found in certain seaweeds, exhibits anti-proliferative properties by promoting dendritic cell maturation and modulating cytokines, ultimately influencing the human immune system. This action involves the activation of macrophages through specific membrane receptors, triggering the production of cytokines like IL-12 and IFN-γ. These cytokines further enhance NK cell and T-cell activation, contributing to cancer cell inhibition.

Studies indicate that fucoidan's ability to inhibit cancer cell growth is linked to the sulfate group of fucose, sulfate content, and molecular weight. Fucoidan derived from Saccharina cichorioides, Fucus evanescens, and Undaria pinnatifida has shown significant suppression of human colon cancer cells while exhibiting minimal cytotoxicity to normal mouse epidermal cells.

However, conflicting results have emerged regarding the correlation between fucoidan and sulfate linkage. Some studies, including Ermakova et al., found that variations in sulfate proportions or the absence of sulfate linkage in fucoidan from certain seaweeds like E. cava, S. hornery, and C. costata did not significantly impact their ability to inhibit human colon cancer cells and melanoma cells.

Moreover, other seaweed-derived secondary metabolites, such as phlorotannins, flavonoids, catechol, carotenoids, quercetin, and myricetin, have demonstrated anticancer activity. Polyphenol-rich Eucheuma cottonii (ECME) showed increased efficacy against estrogen-dependent breast cancer cells compared to estrogen-independent cells. This suggests that the presence of polyphenols in ECME specifically targets cancer-associated receptors and affects gene expression related to cancer cell death.

Epidemiological studies have also indicated a potential link between seaweed consumption and lower incidences of ovarian, breast, and endometrial cancer in the Japanese population compared to other regions globally. This points toward a possible protective effect of seaweed intake against certain types of cancer.

Effect on adipose tissue

Obesity is characterized by an excessive accumulation of fat, particularly in white adipose tissue (WAT), leading to suppressed cytokine secretion in adipose tissue and contributing to various associated disorders like diabetes, hypercholesterolemia, and stroke. The regulation of obesity involves thermogenesis, wherein thermogenic proteins like the uncoupling protein (UCP1, UCP2, and UCP3) families play a significant role in oxidative phosphorylation within brown adipose tissue (BAT). Studies in mice have shown that UCP1 deficiency can lead to increased resistance to obesity.

However, while the presence of brown adipose tissue (BAT) is limited in humans compared to white adipose tissue (WAT), recent research emphasizes the importance of UCP1 expression in WAT for potential anti-obesity therapies. Brown seaweed, such as Undaria pinnatifida, has shown promise in reducing WAT in rats and mice without altering their food intake. Treatment with Undaria lipid-fed rats resulted in a significant reduction in body weight, highlighting the potential of this seaweed in combating obesity.

Moreover, extracts from Undaria pinnatifida, containing fucoxanthin, have been observed to reduce plasma leptin levels and epididymal adipose tissue in mice. Fucoxanthin, found in this extract, notably reduced adipocyte size, fasting blood glucose, and insulin levels in obese rats. Other species like Laminaria japonica and Laminaria ochotensis, containing fucoxanthin, have demonstrated the inhibition of fat absorption and a decrease in serum triglyceride levels in vivo models, showcasing their anti-obesity effects in mice.

Effect on lipid metabolism

Epidemiological studies have highlighted the strong

connection between non-starchy polysaccharides, known as dietary fiber, and lipid metabolism, indicating that diets rich in these polysaccharides promote colon health. Long-term administration of the nutritious seaweed wakame (at 1% in the diet) triggers the peroxisome proliferator-activated receptor pathway, stimulating processes like β-oxidation and gluconeogenesis. This property is attributed to secondary metabolites in seaweed, including ulvan, carrageenan, alginate, fucoidan, and fucoxanthin.

Ulvan derived from Ulva pertusa, with varying molecular weights (U1- 151.6 Da and U2- 28.2 kDa), exhibited anti-hypercholesterolemic effects in hypercholesterolemic rat models. Both U1 and U2 significantly reduced total cholesterol and LDL cholesterol levels by 45.2% and 54.1%, respectively, while elevating serum HDL cholesterol by 22% to 61% compared to a control cereal diet. This underlines how the molecular weight of seaweed polysaccharides influences lipoprotein proportions in lipids. High molecular weight polysaccharides tend to interact with LDL cholesterol, while low molecular weight variants impact triacylglycerol and HDL cholesterol.

Studies by Austin et al. demonstrated that water extracts of A. nodosum contain both polysaccharides and polyphenols, while ethanol extracts primarily consist of a rich polyphenol fraction. The ethanol extract showed more efficient inhibition of lipase, preventing cholesterol absorption. Additionally, concentrates from F. vesiculosus were found to be more potent lipase inhibitors than A. nodosum and Pelvetia canaliculata extracts.

Carrageenan, found in red algae, mimics the texture and sensory quality of lipids, reducing total fat absorption in food. This is attributed to the presence of non-proteinaceous amino acid-like taurine in red algae, which increases the excretion of faecal bile acids and reduces bloodstream cholesterol levels. Seaweed meal inclusion in animal diets increased faecal fat and decreased fat digestibility. Nori and Wakame seaweeds improved colonic fermentation, inhibiting lipid emulsification. Diets incorporating nori and Kombu seaweeds showed lower postprandial lipidemia levels in albino rats. Nori exhibited higher solubility than Kombu, inducing hypocholesterolemic effects due to improved arylesterase activity, impacting lipoprotein metabolism and inhibiting LDL lipid peroxidation. Seaweeds trigger key reactions in lipid metabolism by altering fat emulsification, disrupting micelle formation, modifying lipase enzymes, binding to cholesterol sites, and enhancing colonic bacterial fermentation. Besides polysaccharides, polyphenols, fucoxanthin, and polyunsaturated fatty acids from various seaweeds also influence lipid metabolism through distinct mechanisms.

Applications of Nutraceuticals

Seaweed has become a staple in the food industry, often utilized as a vegetable. Incorporating Chlorella into various food products like pasta and biscuits enhances their nutritional profile. Chlorella and Spirulina are predominantly employed in tablets, capsules, and liquid forms for nutritional supplements owing to their exceptional nutritional content and straightforward cultivation. The edible cyanobacterium Spirulina platensis has garnered global recognition as a food supplement due to its remarkable nutritional value, serving as an abundant source of protein, polyunsaturated fatty acids, and pigments.

Biological medicine

Polysaccharides derived from seaweed exhibit a range of impressive biological activities, including anti-tumor, immunomodulatory, antioxidant, anti-hyperglycemic, anti-cancer, antiviral, anti-fungal, anti-diabetic, anti-hypertensive, anti-inflammatory, UV-protective, and neuroprotective effects. Furthermore, algal hydrogels and hydrocolloids serve as crucial elements in the medical domain, finding extensive application in wound healing, drug delivery, in vitro cell culture, and tissue engineering.

Conclusion and future prospects

Seaweeds are rich reservoirs of functional compounds from secondary metabolisms, including fucoxanthin, phlorotannin, fucoidans, laminarin, carrageenan, alginate, and agar. These compounds find widespread use in food applications due to their various properties, enhancing food quality. While seaweeds have been utilized as functional ingredients in commercial applications as stabilizers, emulsifiers, thickening agents, texture modifiers, and sources of phytochemicals enriched with vitamins and dietary fiber, significant efforts are needed to establish their role and application in health-enhancing foods meant for direct consumption.

Amidst the emergence of the functional food industry and a push for therapeutic food products, seaweed-based products hold immense potential due to their high content of vitamins, fiber, minerals, and omega-3 fatty acids. In vitro studies have demonstrated the efficacy of fortified food products containing seaweed bioactive compounds. However, a key challenge lies in developing new products that resonate with consumers who may be unfamiliar with these offerings. More in-vivo research is necessary to substantiate claims regarding seaweed's potential as an alternative source of health supplements for disease prevention.

Raising public awareness and promoting seaweed as a readily available ingredient with therapeutic effects in daily food consumption is crucial. While numerous studies have evaluated the food, pharmaceutical, and nutraceutical properties of seaweed, further research is essential to understand its safety, toxicity, and environmental impact throughout cultivation, processing, and bioactive extraction for commercial scaling. Stringent testing for contaminants, allergens, heavy metals, and hazardous substances arising from seaweed cultivation or processing is imperative for the development and production of seaweed-based functional food and nutraceutical products, ensuring compliance with safety regulations.Future efforts should focus on sustainable processing of seaweed biomass, aiming for resource efficiency, cleaner pre-treatment techniques to enhance productivity and profitability, and achieving zero waste. A systematic biorefinery approach is crucial to recover a range of commercial compounds from seaweed biomass without leaving behind any waste.

While certain edible seaweeds have been extensively explored for nutraceutical purposes, the vast potential of the sea as a source of nutrient materials for medicinal foods remains largely untapped. Despite efforts to develop new products, industrial-grade products utilizing these nutraceuticals for human health and well-being remain limited. This is primarily due to the necessity for extensive human trials and nutritional intervention studies to establish seaweed as a prime raw material for nutraceuticals at a commercial level. Further research should explore the bio-accessibility and bioavailability of these bioactive compounds for sustained beneficial effects. Additionally, cost-effective cultivation technologies, sustainable biomass processing, and environmentally friendly extraction methods are essential to recover these active molecules from seaweed biomass.

References

1. Bocanegra, S. Bastida, J. Benedi, S. Rodenas, F.J. Sanchez-Muniz, Characteristics and nutritional and cardiovascular-health properties of seaweeds, Journal of Medicinal Food 12(2) (2009) 236-258.

2. G. Rajauria, L. Cornish, F. Ometto, F. E. Msuya, R. Villa, Identification and selection of algae for food, feed, and fuel applications, In Seaweed Sustainability, Academic Press, UK. (2015) pp. 315-345.
3. Y. Miyake, K. Tanaka, H. Okubo, S. Sasaki, M. Arakawa, Seaweed consumption and prevalence of depressive symptoms during pregnancy in Japan: Baseline data from the Kyushu Okinawa Maternal and Child Health Study. BMC Pregnancy and Childbirth 14(1) (2014) 301-307.
4. A. Nanri, T. Mizoue, K. Poudel-Tandukar, M. Noda, M. Kato, K. Kurotani, A. Goto, S. Oba, M. Inoue, S. Tsugane, Dietary patterns and suicide in Japanese adults: the Japan public health center-based prospective study. The British Journal of Psychiatry 203(6) (2013) 422-427.
5. H.J. Lee, H.C. Kim, L. Vitek, C.M. Nam, Algae consumption and risk of type 2 diabetes: Korean National Health and Nutrition Examination Survey in 2005. Journal of Nutritional Science and Vitaminology 56(1) (2010) 13-18.
6. L. Rosenfeld, Discovery and early uses of iodine, Journal of Chemical Education 77(8) (2000) 984.
7. G. Rajauria, B. Foley, N. Abu-Ghannam, Identification and characterization of phenolic antioxidant compounds from brown Irish seaweed Himanthalia elongata using LC-DAD–ESI-MS/MS, Innovative Food Science & Emerging Technologies 37, Part B (2016) 261- 268.
8. J. Teas, S. Vena, D.L. Cone, M. Irhimeh, The consumption of seaweed as a protective factor in the etiology of breast cancer: Proof of principle, Journal of Applied Phycology 25(3) (2013) 771- 779.
9. S.P. Myers, A.M. Mulder, D.G. Baker, S.R. Robinson, M.I. Rolfe, L. Brooks, J.H. Fitton, Effects of fucoidan from Fucus vesiculosus in reducing symptoms of osteoarthritis: A randomized placebo- controlled trial, Biologics: Targets & Therapy 10 (2016) 81- 88.

10. P.R.S. Stephens, C.C. Cirne-Santos, C. de Souza Barros, V.L. Teixeira, L.A.D. Carneiro, L.d.S.C. Amorim, J.S.P. Ocampo, L.R.R. Castello-Branco, I.C.N. de Palmer Paixão, Diterpene from marine brown alga Dictyota friabilis as a potential microbicide against HIV1 in tissue explants, Journal of Applied Phycology 29(2) (2017) 775-780.
11. S. Nagarajan, M. Mathaiyan, Emerging novel anti HIV biomolecules from marine Algae: An overview, Journal of Applied Pharmaceutical Science 5 (2015) 153-158.
12. R.M. Lowenthal, J.H. Fitton, Are seaweed-derived fucoidans possible future anti-cancer agents?, Journal of Applied Phycology 27(5) (2015) 2075-2077.
13. K.W. Lange, J. Hauser, Y. Nakamura, S. Kanaya, Dietary seaweeds and obesity, Food Science and Human Wellness 4(3) (2015) 87-96.
14. Y. Wang, G. Chen, Y. Peng, Y. Rui, X. Zeng, H. Ye, Simulated digestion and fermentation in vitro with human gut microbiota of polysaccharides from Coralline pilulifera, LWT-Food Science and Technology 100 (2019) 167-174.
15. R.G. Abirami, S. Kowsalya, Antidiabetic activity of Ulva fasciata and its impact on carbohydrate metabolism enzymes in alloxan induced diabetic rats, International Journal of Research in Pharmacology and Phytochemistry 3(3) (2013) 136-141.
16. H. Maeda, S. Kanno, M. Kodate, M. Hosokawa, K. Miyashita, Fucoxanthinol, metabolite of fucoxanthin, improves obesity-induced inflammation in adipocyte cells, Marine Drugs 13(8) (2015) 4799-4813.
17. E. Apostolidis, P.D. Karayannakidis, Y.-I. Kwon, C.M. Lee, N.P. Seeram, Seasonal variation of phenolic antioxidant-mediated α-glucosidase inhibition of Ascophyllum nodosum, Plant Foods for Human Nutrition 66(4) (2011) 313-319.

18. K.T. Kim, L.E. Rioux, S.L. Turgeon, Alpha-amylase and alpha-glucosidase inhibition is differentially modulated by fucoidan obtained from Fucus vesiculosus and Ascophyllum nodosum, Phytochemistry 98 (2014) 27-33.

19. K. Iwai, Antidiabetic and Antioxidant Effects of Polyphenols in Brown Alga Ecklonia stolonifera in Genetically Diabetic KK-Ay Mice, Plant Foods for Human Nutrition 63(4) (2008) 163.

20. S.H. Lee, Y.J. Jeon, Anti-diabetic effects of brown algae derived phlorotannins, marine polyphenols through diverse mechanisms, Fitoterapia 86 (2013) 129-136.

21. J. Kellogg, D. Esposito, M.H. Grace, S. Komarnytsky, M.A. Lila, Alaskan seaweeds lower inflammation in RAW 264.7 macrophages and decrease lipid accumulation in 3T3-L1 adipocytes, Journal of Functional Foods 15 (2015) 396-407.

22. S. Ermakova, R. Sokolova, S.-M. Kim, B.-H. Um, V. Isakov, T. Zvyagintseva, Fucoidans from brown seaweeds Sargassum hornery, Eclonia cava, Costaria costata: structural characteristics and anticancer activity, Applied Biochemistry and Biotechnology 164(6) (2011) 841-850.

23. M.T. Ale, H. Maruyama, H. Tamauchi, J.D. Mikkelsen, A.S. Meyer, Fucose-containing sulfated polysaccharides from brown seaweeds inhibit proliferation of melanoma cells and induce apoptosis by activation of caspase-3 in vitro, Marine Drugs 9(12) (2011) 2605-2621.

24. F. Namvar, S. Mohamed, S.G. Fard, J. Behravan, N.M. Mustapha, N.B.M. Alitheen, F. Othman, Polyphenol-rich seaweed (Eucheuma cottonii) extract suppresses breast tumour via hormone modulation and apoptosis induction, Food Chemistry 130(2) (2012) 376-382.

25. N. Mikami, M. Hosokawa, K. Miyashita, H. Sohma, Y.M. Ito, Y. Kokai, Reduction of HbA1c levels by fucoxanthin-enriched akamoku oil possibly involves the thrifty allele of uncoupling protein 1 (UCP1): a

randomised controlled trial in normal-weight and obese Japanese adults, Journal of Nutritional Science 6 (2017) e5-e5.

26. K. Yoshinaga, Y. Nakai, H. Izumi, K. Nagaosa, T. Ishijima, T. Nakano, K. Abe, Oral Administration of Edible Seaweed Undaria Pinnatifida (Wakame) Modifies Glucose and Lipid Metabolism in Rats: A DNA Microarray Analysis, Molecular Nutrition & Food Research 62(12) (2018) 1700828.

27. K. A.Grasa-López, Á. Miliar-García, L. Quevedo-Corona, N. Paniagua-Castro, G. EscalonaCardoso, E. Reyes-Maldonado, M.-E. Jaramillo-Flores, Undaria pinnatifida and Fucoxanthin Ameliorate Lipogenesis and Markers of Both Inflammation and Cardiovascular Dysfunction in an Animal Model of Diet-Induced Obesity, Marine Drugs 14(8) (2016) 148.

28. M.A. Gammone, N. D'Orazio, Anti-obesity activity of the marine carotenoid fucoxanthin, Marine Drugs 13(4) (2015) 2196-2214.

29. S.I. Kang, H.-S. Shin, H.-M. Kim, S.-A. Yoon, S.-W. Kang, J.-H. Kim, H.-C. Ko, S.-J. Kim, Petalonia binghamiae Extract and Its Constituent Fucoxanthin Ameliorate High-Fat Diet-Induced Obesity by Activating AMP-Activated Protein Kinase, Journal of Agricultural and Food Chemistry 60(13) (2012) 3389-3395.

30. Qi, H., Huang, L., Liu, X., Liu, D., Zhang, Q., & Liu, S. (2012). Antihyperlipidemic activity of high sulfate content derivative of polysaccharide extracted from Ulva pertusa (Chlorophyta). Carbohydrate Polymers, 87(2), 1637-1640.

31. Austin, D. Stewart, J.W. Allwood, G.J. McDougall, Extracts from the edible seaweed, Ascophyllum nodosum, inhibit lipase activity in vitro: contributions of phenolic and polysaccharide components, Food & Function 9(1) (2018) 502-510.

32. P.I. Chater, M. Wilcox, P. Cherry, A. Herford, S. Mustar, H. Wheater, I. Brownlee, C. Seal, J. Pearson, Inhibitory activity of extracts of Hebridean brown seaweeds on lipase activity, Journal of Applied Phycology 28(2) (2016) 1303-1313.
33. Ganesan, A. R., Shanmugam, M., & Bhat, R. (2019). Quality enhancement of chicken sausage by semi-refined carrageenan. Journal of Food Processing and Preservation, e13988.
34. T.H. Yang, H.-T. Yao, M.-T. Chiang, Red algae (Gelidium amansii) hot-water extract ameliorates lipid metabolism in hamsters fed a high-fat diet, Journal of Food and Drug Analysis 25(4) (2017) 931-938.
35. P. Matanjun, S. Mohamed, K. Muhammad, N.M. Mustapha, Comparison of Cardiovascular Protective Effects of Tropical Seaweeds, Kappaphycus alvarezii, Caulerpa lentillifera, and Sargassum polycystum, on High-Cholesterol/High-Fat Diet in Rats, Journal of Medicinal Food 13(4) (2010) 792-800.
36. J. Kellogg, D. Esposito, M.H. Grace, S. Komarnytsky, M.A. Lila, Alaskan seaweeds lower inflammation in RAW 264.7 macrophages and decrease lipid accumulation in 3T3-L1 adipocytes, Journal of Functional Foods 15 (2015) 396-407.
37. M.W.-A. Airanthi, N. Sasaki, S. Iwasaki, N. Baba, M. Abe, M. Hosokawa, K. Miyashita, Effect of brown seaweed lipids on fatty acid composition and lipid hydroperoxide levels of mouse liver, Journal of Agricultural and Food Chemistry 59(8) (2011) 4156-4163.
38. K. Ruqqia, V. Sultana, J. Ara, S. Ehteshamul-Haque, M. Athar, Hypolipidaemic potential of seaweeds in normal, triton-induced and high-fat diet-induced hyperlipidaemic rats, Journal of Applied Phycology 27(1) (2015) 571-579.

Chapter-15

Nutraceutical Properties of Lotus

Introduction
The lotus plant, particularly the 'sacred blue lotus' (Nymphaea caerulea), held significant cultural and religious importance in ancient times along the Nile River in Egypt. It was revered by Pharaonic Egyptians, depicted widely in their architectural motifs, and later spread to Assyria, Persia, India, and China. Introduced to Western Europe in 1787 under Sir Joseph Banks' patronage, it became a prevalent feature in modern botanical gardens globally.

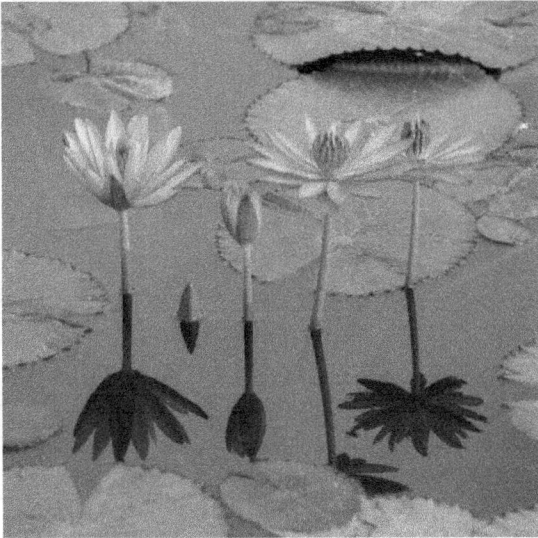

Lotus plants are found abundantly in Australia, China, India, Iran, and Japan, with a history spanning over a thousand years in Chinese cultivation. In China, it was cultivated extensively as an industrial crop, occupying over 40,000 hectares in 1999. India boasts widespread lotus growth, even in Himalayan lakes at altitudes reaching up to 1400 meters.

The seeds of the lotus, known as 'kamal gatta' in Indian markets, serve as both a vegetable and a raw material for Ayurvedic preparations. Renowned for their health benefits, lotus seeds and roots are considered popular health foods. Extracts from lotus, like the alkaloid liensinine, exhibit effectiveness in treating arrhythmia.

Botanically classified under Nelumbonaceae, Nelumbo nucifera, or the lotus, goes by various common names such as Indian lotus, Chinese water lily, and sacred lotus. It is a perennial, large, rhizomatous aquatic herb characterized by elongated, creeping stems with nodal roots. The leaves are membranous, peltate, and cup-shaped, growing over 60-90 centimeters. Petioles are lengthy, rough, and feature small prickles. Its flowers, sweet-scented and white to rosy, are solitary and hermaphroditic, ranging from 10-25 centimeters in diameter. The ripe carpels are ovoid, around 12 millimeters long and glabrous, while the fruits resemble ovoid achenes. Lotus seeds are hard, black, and ovoid in shape.

Nutritional value

The tender rhizomes, stems, and leaves of the lotus plant are edible and can be prepared in various ways: cooked alongside other vegetables, soaked in syrup, or pickled in vinegar. Lotus rhizomes, constituting 1.7% protein, 0.1% fat, 9.7% carbohydrates, and 1.1% ash, impart a mild flavor and are extensively used in Chinese recipes. When cooked, lotus stems resemble the taste of beets. In Vietnam, the lotus stem, containing calcium, iron, and zinc (6, 2.4, 0.2 mg/100 g respectively), is commonly used in salads.

In traditional practices, lotus leaves are employed as a remedy for summer heat syndrome in Japan and China, and in China specifically for managing obesity. The petals are often floated in soups or utilized as a decorative garnish, while the stamens contribute to tea flavoring. Egyptian lotus seeds, with a crude protein content of 14.8%, contain bitter green embryos that are typically removed before selling in markets. These seeds can be popped like popcorn, ground into powder for consumption, or incorporated into bread making. Roasted lotus seeds serve as a coffee substitute and contain notable quantities of saponins, phenolics, and carbohydrates.

The nutritional composition of lotus seeds includes 10.5% moisture, 10.6-15.9% protein, 1.93-2.8% crude fat, 70-72.17% carbohydrates, 2.7% crude fiber, 3.9-4.5% ash, with an energy content of 348.45 cal/100 g. Lotus seeds are also rich in essential minerals such as chromium (0.0042%), sodium (1%), potassium (28.5%), calcium (22.1%), magnesium (9.2%), copper (0.0463%), zinc (0.084%), manganese (0.356%), and iron (0.199%).

Pharmaceutical value

Traditional knowledge

The traditional knowledge surrounding the lotus plant highlights its diverse medicinal uses. The entire plant exhibits astringent, emollient, diuretic, and sudorific properties and is known for its antifungal, antipyretic, and cardiotonic effects. Various parts of the lotus plant are employed in treating diarrhea, tissue inflammation, and aiding in hemostasis.

The rhizome extract, containing asteroidal triterpenoids, exhibits anti-diabetic and anti-inflammatory properties. Rhizomes are utilized for treating conditions such as pharyngopathy, pectoralgia, spermatorrhoea, leucoderma, smallpox, diarrhea, dysentery, and cough. The stem is included in indigenous Ayurvedic remedies as a diuretic, anthelmintic, and treatment for conditions like strangury, vomiting, leprosy, skin diseases, and nervous exhaustion.

Young leaves combined with sugar are used to address rectal prolapse, while boiling the leaves with Mimosa pudica in

221

goat's milk is employed to treat diarrhea. Leaf paste is applied to the body during fever and inflammatory skin conditions. The leaves are considered an effective remedy for bleeding disorders such as hematemesis, epistaxis, hemoptysis, hematuria, and metrorrhagia. Lotus leaves also exhibit therapeutic potential in treating hyperlipidemia in rodents, acting as diuretics and astringents, aiding in the treatment of fever, sweating, and strangury, and serving as a styptic.

The leaves and flowers are utilized to treat various bleeding disorders, and flower consumption is recommended to enhance conception. Lotus flowers are employed in managing conditions such as diarrhea, cholera, fever, hepatopathy, and hyperdipsia. In folk medicine, lotus seeds are utilized to treat tissue inflammation, cancer, skin diseases, leprosy, and as a general diuretic for children. The fruits and seeds possess astringent properties and are used in addressing hyperdipsia, dermatopathy, halitosis, menorrhagia, leprosy, and fever.

Seed powder combined with honey is effective in treating cough, while roots mixed with ghee, milk, and gold are believed to promote strength, virility, and intellect. Lotus seeds are recognized for their rich antimicrobial properties. The embryo of lotus seeds is used in traditional Chinese medicine known as 'Lian Zi Xin', which aids in addressing nervous disorders, insomnia, high fevers accompanied by restlessness, and cardiovascular diseases like hypertension and arrhythmia.

Alkaloids and flavonoids

Lotus alkaloids have the ability to widen blood vessels, thereby lowering blood pressure. The leaves possess a bittersweet taste and contain various flavonoids and alkaloids. The embryos found within the lotus seeds contain a small amount of alkaloids known for their antispasmodic effects on the intestines, providing relief from diarrhea. Specifically, these embryos contain an alkaloid called isoquinoline, which acts as a sedative and antispasmodic agent while benefiting the heart. This compound is effective in dispelling pathogenic heat from the heart and mitigating spontaneous bleeding due to heat.

Lotus seeds are rich in various phytochemicals, particularly alkaloids such as dauricine, lotusine, nuciferine, pronuciferine, liensinine, isoliensinine, roemerine, nelumbine, and neferine. Dauricine and neferine are known to block the transmembrane currents of Na+, K+, and Ca2+ in cardiac cells. Neferine, functioning as an anti-arrhythmic agent, significantly inhibits rabbit platelet aggregation.

Lim et al. (2006) conducted research on the rat lens aldose reductase (RLAR), an enzyme associated with the polyol pathway in diabetes, and its inhibitory constituents found in the stamens of N. nucifera. The methanol extract from these stamens showed inhibitory effects on RLAR. Thirteen flavonoids and seven glycosides of flavonoids were isolated from lotus plants, along with four non-flavonoid compounds. Among these isolated flavonoids, those containing 3-O-alpha-l-rhamnopyranosyl-(1 → 6)-beta-d-glucopyranoside groups in their C rings—such as kaempferol 3-O-alpha-l-rhamnopyranosyl-(1→6)-beta-d-glucopyranoside and isorhamnetin 3-O-alpha-l-rhamnopyranosyl-(1→6)-beta-d-glucopyranoside—demonstrated the highest RLAR inhibitory activity in vitro, with an IC50 of 5.6 and 9.0 μM, respectively.

Antioxidants

Ushimaru et al. (2001) delved into the changes in antioxidative enzymes within N. nucifera seedlings responding to oxygen deficiency during germination under water conditions. They found that seedlings germinated under submerged darkness (SD) exhibited lower activity in superoxide dismutase, dehydroascorbate reductase, and glutathione reductase compared to those germinated in air and darkness (AD). However, ascorbate peroxidase activity was higher in SD seedlings than in AD seedlings. On the other hand, catalase and monodehydroascorbate reductase activities in SD seedlings were nearly equivalent to those in AD seedlings. Additionally, leaf stalk extracts demonstrated antipyretic effects, while antioxidant properties were identified in leaves and stamens. Lotus seed extracts were found to possess hepatoprotective, free radical scavenging, and antifertility properties (Sohn et al., 2003).

Yen et al. (2006) reported on the free radical scavenging and protective effects of lotus seed extracts (LSE) against reactive nitrogen, sodium nitroprusside (SNP), and peroxynitrite-induced cytotoxicity and DNA damage in macrophage RAW 264.7 cell lines. Extracts obtained via water (LSWE), ethyl acetate (LSEAE), and hexane (LSHE) were assessed for their inhibitory effects. These extracts demonstrated inhibitory effects on nitric oxide accumulation in LPS-activated RAW 264.7 cells. The extracts showed a dose-dependent inhibitory effect on nitric oxide accumulation upon SNP decomposition. LSWEAE exhibited the highest potency in inhibitory activity, followed by LSWE and LSHE. These extracts also showed no significant difference in DNA damage between control and sample groups in RAW 264.7 cells. Moreover, these extracts demonstrated the ability to inhibit DNA damage induced by SNP. LSWE, LSEAE, and LSHE at 0.2 mg/ml exhibited 63%, 59%, and 38% inhibition, respectively, of peroxynitrite-induced DNA damage in macrophage RAW 264.7 cells. Furthermore, these extracts proved to be potent peroxynitrite scavengers in preventing tyrosine nitration, with LSWE, LSEAE, and LSHE at 0.2 mg/ml showing 29.0%, 21.0%, and 8.0% inhibition, respectively, against control values.

Rai et al. (2006) explored the antioxidant activity of hydro-alcoholic extracts of lotus seeds using both in vitro and in vivo models. The extract displayed strong free radical scavenging activity, demonstrated by low IC50 values (16.12 μg/ml) in 1,1-diphenyl-2-picryl hydrazyl, comparable to rutin (IC50, 18.95 μg/ml). In the nitric oxide method, the extract exhibited higher activity (IC50, 84.86 μg/ml) than the standard rutin (IC50, 152.17 μg/ml). No signs of acute toxicity were observed up to an oral dose of 1,000 mg/kg body weight in Swiss Albino mice.

Ling et al. (2005) conducted groundbreaking research on procyanidins in the non-edible parts of lotus. They extracted procyanidins from lotus pods with a purity of up to 98% in Me2CO-H2O and purified them using Sephadex LH-20 column chromatography. The ESI-MS analysis revealed a distribution of molecular weights ranging from 291 to 1155, primarily consisting of monomers, dimers, and tetramers of procyanidins, with a higher proportion of dimers, catechin, and epicatechin base units. The extract was a light red-brown amorphous powder. Spectrometric quantification demonstrated that the extract contained 90.7% total polyphenols and 98.3% procyanidin. The scavenging effect of lotus pod procyanidin on superoxide free radicals (O2 −) resulted in an IC50 of 17.6 mg/l, equivalent to 0.3 mg/l vitamin C. The extract also demonstrated scavenging effects on ·OH. At a concentration of 0.1%, procyanidin extract exhibited a strong antioxidant activity similar to butylated hydroxytoluene (BHT) in inhibiting the auto-oxidation of lard after eight days. This data indicated that the procyanidin partially inhibited the autoxidation of lard, with 0.1% procyanidin showing robust antioxidant properties.

Antisteroids

Gupta et al. (1996) detailed the antisteroidogenic effects of N. nucifera seed extract in both the testis and ovary of rats. Administering fractions of the petroleum ether extract orally to sexually immature female rats and mature male rats over a 15-day period resulted in a delay in sexual maturation among pre-pubertal female rats, indicated by delayed vaginal opening and first estrus (cornified smear), and a reduction in sperm count and motility in mature male rats. These treatments led to increased accumulation of cholesterol and ascorbic acid, while reducing delta-5-3-beta-hydroxysteroid dehydrogenase and glucose-6-phosphate dehydrogenase activity in the ovary and testis, indicating suppression of steroid genesis in both organs.

Antipyretic Properties

Chopra et al. (1958) highlighted the antipyretic potential of N. nucifera. Similarly, Sinha et al. (2000) reported the antipyretic effects of ethanol extracts from lotus stalks, showing a significant reduction in body temperature in both normal conditions and yeast-induced pyrexia in rats. The extract lowered body temperature for up to 3 hours post-administration at 200 mg/kg, and up to 6 hours at 400 mg/kg. In yeast-induced fever, doses of the extract exhibited dose-dependent reductions in body temperature for up to 4 hours, comparable to paracetamol, the standard antipyretic agent (150 mg/kg).

Anticancerous Effects

Liu et al. (2004) found that ethanolic extracts of lotus inhibited cell proliferation and cytokine production in primary human peripheral blood mononuclear cells activated by phytohemagglutinin, a specific mitogen for T lymphocytes. Additionally, Liu et al. (2006) explored the effects of (S)-armepavine, a compound in lotus, in suppressing T cell proliferation. In a study on mice with systemic lupus erythematosus (SLE), (S)-armepavine treatment resulted in a marked decrease in lymphadenopathy and prolonged the lifespan of the mice. It also significantly reduced the production of T lymphocyte-mediated cytokines, specifically IL-2 and IFN-γ, in both mice and human peripheral blood mononuclear cells. This indicated that (S)-armepavine could be considered as an immunomodulator for managing autoimmune diseases like SLE.

Antiviral Properties

Kashiwada et al. (2005) isolated anti-HIV compounds, including benzylisoquinoline alkaloids and flavonoids, from lotus leaves. These compounds demonstrated potent anti-HIV activities, with (-)-1(S)-norcoclaurine and quercetin 3-O-b-D-glucuronide showing particularly strong effects. Other alkaloids such as liensinine, negferine, and isoliensinine, along with nuciferine, exhibited substantial anti-HIV activities as well. Additionally, ethanolic extracts of lotus seeds were found to suppress replication of herpes simplex type 1 (HSV-1), even in cases of acyclovir-resistant HSV-1 strains, as observed by Kuo et al. (2005). The study highlighted NN-B-5, extracted from the bioactive NN-B fraction obtained from butanol, as having the highest suppressive activity against HSV-1 replication, indicating its potential to curb acyclovir-resistant HSV-1 propagation.

Ono et al. (2006) investigated the anti-obesity effects of lotus N. nucifera leaf extract (NNE) in mice and rats. The leaf extract showed concentration-dependent inhibition of α-amylase and lipase activities, boosting lipid metabolism, and enhancing the expression of UCP3 mRNA in C2C12 myotubes over five weeks of treatment. NNE also demonstrated strong inhibition of lipase compared to α-amylase activity, both in vitro and in vivo. In obese mice fed a high-fat diet, the extract prevented increases in body weight, parametrial adipose tissue weight, and liver triacylglycerol levels. Moreover, there was an inclination toward higher UCP3 mRNA expression in skeletal muscle.

Future Perspectives

The exploration of lotus seeds for bioprospecting shows

promising potential as an alternative protein source and pharmaceutical reservoir. However, detailed studies on potential long-term toxic effects from lotus seed consumption are needed. While the nutraceutical value of lotus seeds is established, further research on identifying additional beneficial compounds could enhance their health-promoting properties. Addressing issues related to microbial contamination and spoilage in lotus seeds, including examining contaminants, spoilage microflora (such as bacteria and fungi), their toxins, and control measures, would be crucial for wider acceptance and use. Considering the nutraceutical advantages, combining lotus seed flour with other nutrient-rich legumes (like soybeans) or millets (such as finger millet) could create cost-effective protein-rich health supplements, aiding in combating malnutrition and specific health conditions.

References
1. Anonymous. (1966). The Wealth of India - A Dictionary of Indian Raw Materials. Volume 7, Council of Scientific Industrial Research, New Delhi, India.
2. Anonymous. (1992). The Wealth of India. Volume 3, Council of Scientific Industrial Research, New Delhi, India.
3. Arunyanart, S. and Chaitrayagun, M. (2005). Induction of somatic embryogenesis in lotus (Nelumbo nucifera Gaertn.). Scientia Horticulturae 105: 411-420.
4. Chen, Yi., Fan, G., Wu, H., Wu, Y. and Mitchell A. (2007). Separation, identification and rapid determination of liensine, isoliensinine and neferine from embryo of the seed of Nelumbo nucifera Gaertn. by liquid chromatography coupled to diode array detector and tandem mass spectrometry. Journal of Pharmaceutical and Biomedical Analysis 43: 99-104.

5. Chinese Materia Medica (1977). Jiangsu New Medical College, Peoples Publishing House, Shanghai, China.
6. Chopra, R.N., Nayar, S.L. and Chopra, I.C. (1956). Glossary of Indian Medicinal Plants. Council of Scientific Industrial Research, New Delhi, India.
7. Chopra, R. N., Chopra, I. C. and Handa, K.L. (1958). Indigenous Drugs of India. 2nd Edition, U.N. Dhur and Sons Pvt. Ltd., Calcutta, India.
8. Facciola, S. (1990). Cornucopia: A Source Book of Edible Plants. Kampong Publications, California. Famurewa, J.A.V. and Raji, A.O. (2005). Parameters affecting milling qualities of undefatted soybeans (Glycine max L. Merill) (1), Selected thermal treatment. International Journal of Food Engineering 1: 1-9.
9. FAO (1994). The State of Food and Agriculture. FAO agricultural series # 27, FAO/UN, Rome.
10. Furukawa, H., Yang, T.H. and Lin, T.J. (1965). Effect of Nelumbo nucifera rhizomeextract on blood sugar level in rats. Yakugaku Zasshi 85: 472-475.
11. Gupta, M., Mazumder, U.K., Mukhopadhyay, R.K. and Sarkar, S. (1996). Antisteroidogenic effect of the seed extract of Nelumbo nucifera in the testis and the ovary of the rat. Indian Journal of Pharmaceutical Science 58: 236-242.
12. Hedrick, U.P. (1972). Sturtevant's Edible Plants of the World. (ed Hedrick. U.P.). Dover Publications, New York.
13. Ibrahim, N. and El-Eraqy, W. (1996). Protein content and amino acid composition of Nelumbo nucifera seeds and its evaluation as hypoglycaemic agent. Egyptian journal of pharmaceutical sciences 37: 635-641
14. Indrayan, A.K., Sharma, S., Durgapal, D., Kumar, N. and Kumar, M. (2005). Determination of nutritive value and analysis of mineral elements for some medicinally valued plants from Uttaranchal. Current Science 89: 1252-1255.

15. Jung, H.A., Kim, J.E., Chung, H.Y.A. and Choi, J.S. (2003). Antioxidant principles of Nelumbo nucifera stamens. Archives of Pharmacological Research 26: 279-285.

16. Kashiwada, Y., Aoshima, A., Ikeshiro, Y., Yuh-Pan, Chen, Furukawa, H., Itoigawa, M., Fujioka, T., Mihashi, K., Cosentino, M.L., Susan, L. Morris-Natschke and Lee, K.H. (2005). Anti-HIV benzylisoquinoline alkaloids and flavonoids from the leaves of Nelumbo nucifera and structure-activity correlations with related alkaloids. Bioorganic Medicinal Chemistry 13: 443-448.

17. Komatsu, E., Tsukahara, A., Amagaya, H., Okazawa, N., Noguchi, T. and Okuyama, T. (1975). Lotus. In: The Cultivation and Management in Aquatic Vegetables (ed Izaki, M.).

18. Ie-No-Hikari Kyokai Press, Tokyo, 9-94. Kuo, Y.-C., Lin, Y.-L., Liu C.-P. and Tsai, W.-J. (2005). Herpes simplex virus type 1 propagation in HeLa cells interrupted by Nelumbo nucifera. Journal of Biomedical Science 12: 1021-1034.

19. La Cour, B., Molgaard, P. and Yi, Z. (1995). Traditional Chinese medicine in treatment of hyperlipidaemia. Journal of Ethnopharmacology 46: 125-129. Li, G.R., Qian, J.Q. and Lu, F.H. (1990). Effects of neferine on heart electromechanical activity in anaesthetized cats. Zhongguo Yao Li Xue Bao 11: 158-161.

20. Lim, S.S., Jung, Y.J., Hyun, S.K., Lee, Y.S. and Choi, J.S. (2006). Rat lens aldose reductase inhibitory constituents of Nelumbo nucifera stamens. Pyhtotherapy Research 20: 825- 830.

21. Ling, Z.Q., Xie, B.J. and Yang, E.L. (2005). Isolation, characterization, and determination of antioxidative activity of oligomeric procyanidins from the seedpod of Nelumbo nucifera Gaertn. Journal of Agricultural and Food Chemistry 53: 2441-2445.

22. Liu, C.P., Tsai, W.J., Lin, Y.L., Liao, J.F., Chen, C.F. and Kuo, Y.C. (2004). The extracts from Nelumbo nucifera suppress cell cycle progression, cytokine genes expression, and cell proliferation in human peripheral blood mononuclear cells. Life Sciences 75: 699-716.
23. Liu, C.-P., Tsai, W.-J., Shen, C.-C., Lin, Y.-L, Liao, J.-F., Chen, C.-F. and Kuo, Y.-C. (2006). Inhibition of (S)-armepavine from Nelumbo nucifera on autoimmune disease of MRL/MpJ-lpr/lpr mice. European Journal of Pharmacology 531: 270-279.
24. Michaelsen, K.F. and Henrik, F. (1998). Complementary feeding: A global perspective. Nutrition 14: 763-766.
25. Mukherjee, P.K. (2002). Quality Control of Herbal Drugs - An Approach to Evaluation of Botanicals. 1st Edition, Business Horizons, New Delhi, India.
26. Mukherjee, P.K., Giri, S.N., Saha, K., Pal, M. and Saha, B.P. (1995). Antifungal screening of Nelumbo nucifera (Nymphaeaceae) rhizome extract. Indian Journal of Microbiology 35: 327-330.
27. Mukherjee, P.K., Saha, K. and Saha, B.P. (1997a). Effect of Nelumbo nucifera rhizome extract on blood sugar level in rats. Journal of Ethnopharmacology 58: 207-213.
28. Mukherjee, P.K., Saha, K., Das, J., Pal, M. and Saha, B.P. (1997b). Studies on the antiinflammatory activity of rhizomes of Nelumbo nucifera. Planta Medica 63: 367-369.
29. Nadkarni, A.K. (1982). The Indian Materia Medica. Volume 1, Popular Prakashan Pvt. Ltd., Bombay, India.
30. Ogle, B.M., Dao, H.T.A., Mulokozi, G. and Hambraeus, L. (2001). Micronutrient composition and nutritional importance of gathered vegetables in Vietnam. International Journal of Food Science and Nutrition 52: 485-499.
31. Onishi, E., Yamada, K., Yamada, T., Kaji, K., Inoue, H., Seyama, Y. and Yamashita, S. (1984). Comparative

effects of crude drugs on serum lipids. Chemical & Pharmaceutical Bulletin 32: 646-650.

32. Ono, Y., Hattori, E., Fukaya, Y., Imai, S. and Ohizumi, Y. (2006). Antiobesity effect of Nelumbo nucifera leaves extract in mice and rats. Journal of Ethnopharmacology 106: 238-244.

33. Ou, M. (1989). Chinese-English Manual of Common-used in Traditional Chinese Medicine. Joint Publishing Co. Ltd., Hong Kong.

34. Phillips, R. and Rix, M. (1995). Vegetables. Macmillan Reference Books, London.

35. Polunin, O. and Stainton, A. (1984). Flowers of the Himalayas. Oxford University Press, New Delhi, India.

36. Qian, J.Q. (2002). Cardiovascular pharmacological effects of bisbenzylisoquinoline alkaloid derivatives. Acta Pharmacologica Sinica 23: 1086-1092.

37. Rai, S., Wahile, A., Mukherjee, K., Saha, B.P. and Mukherjee, P.K. (2006). Antioxidant activity of Nelumbo nucifera (sacred lotus) seeds. Journal of Ethonopharmacology 104: 322-327.

38. Ramsbottom, J. (1942). Recent work on germination. Nature 149: 658.

39. Reid, B.E. (1977). Famine Foods of the Chiu-Huang Pen-ts'ao. Southern Materials Centre, Taipei.

40. Shoji, N., Umeyama, A., Saito, N., Iuchi, A., Takemoto, T., Kajiwara, A., Ohizumi, Y. (1987). Asimilobine and lirinidine, serotonergic receptor antagonists, from Nelumbo nucifera. Journal of Natural Products 50: 773-774.

41. Sinha, S., Mukherjee, P.K., Mukherjee, K., Pal, M., Mandal, S.C. and Saha1, B.P. (2000). Evaluation of antipyretic potential of Nelumbo nucifera stalk extract. Phytotherapy Research 14: 272-274.

42. Sohn, D.H., Kim, Y.C., Oh, S.H., Park, E.J., Li, X. and Lee, B.H. (2003). Hepatoprotective and free radical

Food Pharmacies : A Guide to Nutraceutical Riches

scavenging effects of Nelumbo nucifera. Phytomedicine 10: 165-69.

43. Tanaka, T. (1976). Tanaka's Cyclopaedia of Edible Plants of the World. Keigaku Publishing Co., Tokyo.

44. Tomita, M., Furukawa, H. and Yang, T.H. (1961). Alkaloids of Nelumbo nucifera I. Yakugaku Zasshi 81: 469-473.

45. Ushimaru, T., Kanematsu, S., Katayama, M. and Tsuji, H. (2001). Antioxidative enzymes in seedlings of Nelumbo nucifera germinated under water. Physiologia Plantarum 112: 39- 46.

46. Wang, J., Hu, X., Yin, W. and Cai, H. (1991). Alkaloids of Plumula nelumbinis. Zhongguo Zhong Yao Za Zhi 16: 673-675.

47. Wu, M.J., Wang, L., Weng, C.Y. and Yen, J.H. (2003). Antioxidant activity of methanol extract of the lotus leaf (Nelumbo nucifera Gertn.). American Journal of Chinese Medicine 31: 687-698.

48. Yen, G-C., Duh, P-D., Su, H-J., Yeha, C-T. and Wu, C-H. (2006). Scavenging effects of lotus seed extracts on reactive nitrogen species. Food Chemistry 94: 596-602. Yu, J. and Hu, W.S. (1997). Effects of neferine on platelet aggregation in rabbits. Yaoxue Xuebao 32: 1-4.

Chapter- 16

Nutraceuticals Extraction : Techniques, Advancements and Challenges

Introduction
Nutraceuticals, derived from natural sources, have garnered considerable attention for their potential health benefits. Extraction procedures play a pivotal role in isolating these bioactive compounds, facilitating their application in pharmaceuticals, functional foods, dietary supplements, and cosmetics. This review explores the diverse methodologies employed in nutraceutical extraction, recent advancements in extraction techniques, challenges encountered, and future directions in this field.

Methodologies for Nutraceuticals Extraction

Solvent-Based Extraction Techniques
Solvent extraction remains a prevalent method due to its versatility. Utilizing solvents like ethanol, methanol, water, or their mixtures, this technique dissolves and extracts a broad spectrum of compounds from various natural sources. Its efficiency in obtaining crude extracts containing bioactive compounds makes it a widely used and adaptable approach.

Innovative Extraction Technologies
Advancements in extraction methodologies have led to the development of innovative techniques:

Supercritical Fluid Extraction (SFE) : Leveraging supercritical fluids like carbon dioxide under specific conditions, SFE enables selective extraction while preserving compound integrity. This method is particularly advantageous for heat-sensitive compounds, ensuring the extraction of delicate bioactive substances.

Ultrasound-Assisted Extraction : Ultrasonic waves enhance mass transfer rates, disrupting cell walls and expediting the release of bioactive compounds. This technology offers high efficiency and reduced extraction times, contributing to a more sustainable extraction process.

Microwave-Assisted Extraction (MAE) : By utilizing microwave energy, MAE accelerates the extraction process by increasing temperature and pressure within the extraction vessel. This method aids in cell disruption, facilitating compound release and reducing extraction times.

Factors Influencing Extraction Efficiency

Numerous factors influence the efficiency of nutraceutical extraction :

Source Material Selection: Variations in raw materials, including different plant parts or marine organisms, significantly impact the types and concentrations of bioactive compounds obtained.

Particle Size and Surface Area : Finer particle size increases surface area, enhancing contact between the material and solvent, thus improving extraction efficiency.

Extraction Parameters : Temperature, pressure, extraction time, and the ratio of solvent to material play crucial roles in determining extraction efficiency and selectivity.

Challenges and Future Directions

Despite significant advancements, several challenges persist in nutraceutical extraction:

Standardization : Ensuring consistent quality and potency of nutraceutical extracts remains challenging due to variations in raw materials and extraction methods. Standardization protocols are imperative for quality control and reliability.

Sustainabilit : Eco-friendly extraction techniques, employing greener solvents and reducing energy consumption, are essential for minimizing the environmental impact of extraction processes.

Technological Advancements : Ongoing research focuses on developing and improving extraction technologies to enhance efficiency, yield, and specificity. Innovations in extraction methodologies continue to expand the repertoire of extracted nutraceutical compounds.

Conclusion

The extraction of nutraceuticals from natural sources encompasses diverse methodologies, each with its advantages and limitations. Advancements in extraction techniques, coupled with a deeper understanding of plant chemistry, continue to refine these processes. Sustainable and innovative approaches are essential to ensure consistent quality, enhance efficiency, and expand the range of extracted bioactive compounds. As these methods evolve, nutraceuticals will continue to play a pivotal role in promoting human health and wellness across various industries.

References

1. Zhang, Zhonghua, et al. "Ultrasound-assisted extraction of polysaccharides from mulberry leaves." Ultrasonics Sonochemistry, vol. 17, no. 5, 2010, pp. 921-925.
2. Chemat, Farid, and Giancarlo Cravotto. "Microwave-assisted extraction for bioactive compounds." Microwave-Assisted Extraction for Bioactive Compounds, Springer, 2013, pp. 1-22.
3. Sharma, Om Prakash, et al. "A review on microwave-assisted extraction as a green method for food and natural products." Green Chemistry Letters and Reviews, vol. 10, no. 2, 2017, pp. 113-127.
4. Khaw, Kooi-Yeong, et al. "Supercritical fluid extraction of bioactive compounds from plants and algae." Critical Reviews in Food Science and Nutrition, vol. 57, no. 11, 2017, pp. 2453-2468.

5. Patel, Jignesh, et al. "Current trends in natural preservatives for extending shelf life of fresh meat products." Journal of Food Science and Technology, vol. 54, no. 11, 2017, pp. 3387-3399.
6. Dulf, Francisc, et al. "Solvent extraction of bioactive compounds from plant materials." Engineering Aspects of Food Biotechnology, CRC Press, 2018, pp. 119-142.
7. Costa, Elina Bastos, et al. "Nutraceuticals and functional foods: Trends in extraction procedures of bioactive compounds." Comprehensive Reviews in Food Science and Food Safety, vol. 18, no. 3, 2019, pp. 664-677.
8. Barba, Francisco J., et al. "Current applications and new opportunities for the use of pulsed electric fields in food science and industry." Food Research International, vol. 77, Part 4, 2015, pp. 773-798.
9. Pandey, Abhay Kumar, et al. "Advances in application of ultrasound in food processing: A review." Ultrasonics Sonochemistry, vol. 34, 2017, pp. 410-419.
10. Chemat, Farid, and Giancarlo Cravotto. "Green extraction of natural products: Concept and principles." International Journal of Molecular Sciences, vol. 13, no. 7, 2012, pp. 8615-8627

Chapter-17

Regulatory Aspects of Nutraceuticals

Introduction

Nutraceuticals, a burgeoning category of bioactive compounds derived from food sources, have gained immense popularity for their potential to promote health and well-being beyond the scope of basic nutrition. These products, encompassing dietary supplements, functional foods, herbal extracts, and other naturally-derived compounds, bridge the gap between conventional foods and pharmaceuticals. As consumers seek holistic approaches to health and preventive care, the nutraceutical industry has witnessed exponential growth, presenting both opportunities and challenges in the realm of regulation.

The regulatory landscape surrounding nutraceuticals is a complex tapestry, with varying frameworks and guidelines established by different countries and regions. This intricacy arises from the diverse natures of these products, which can contain multiple active components and offer a wide range of health claims. Governments and regulatory bodies worldwide have grappled with defining and categorizing nutraceuticals, harmonizing regulations across borders, and ensuring consumer safety while supporting innovation and market growth.

This chapter aims to explore the regulatory aspects of nutraceuticals, shedding light on the intricate systems governing these products in various parts of the world. It delves into the definitions and categorizations used by different countries, the registration and approval requirements for market entry, labeling guidelines and health claims substantiation, safety assessments, and the challenges faced by regulatory authorities. By comprehending the regulatory landscape, manufacturers, consumers, and healthcare professionals can make informed decisions about the production, sale, and utilization of nutraceuticals.

Th e regulatory framework of nutraceuticals in India needs attention from the relevant authorities. Globally, the regulatory authorities are aware of changing needs of consumers and proactively protect consumers by amending existing laws to accommodate changes but in India old laws such as Prevention of Food adulteration Act, 1954, which regulates packaged foods, still exist for manufacturers. In addition, they need to abide by many other cumbersome laws such as:

Standards of Weights and Measures Act, 1976, and the Standards of Weights and Measures

- (Packaged Commodities) Rules, 1977 (SWMA)
- Infant Milk Substitutes, Feeding bottles and infant foods (regulation of production, Supply and Distribution) Act, 1992 with Rules, 1993 (IMS)
- Edible Oils Packaging (Regulations) Order,1998
- Fruit Products Order 1955 (FPO)
- Meat product Order 1973
- Milk and Milk Products Order 1992
- Vegetable Oils Products (Regulation) Order 1998 (VOP)
- Atomic Energy Act, 1962 and Atomic Energy(Control or irradiation of Food) Rules 1996
- Consumer Protection Act 1986 and the Consumer Protection (Amendment) Act, 2002 and Rules 1987
- Environment Protection Act, 1986 and Rules 1986
- Agricultural Produce (Grading and Marking) Act, 1937 (as amended up to 1986) and 49
- General Grading and Marking Rules 1986 and 1988 (AG Mark)
- Bureau of Indian Standards (BIS) Act 1986

Further, there is lack of clarity in classifying functional foods and Nutraceuticals. Th is causes confusion amongst the regulators. At times, the drug regulators are tempted to classify these products as drugs. Th is has resulted in trouble for genuine manufacturers. Th e revolutionary step to introduce Food Safety and Standards Act will replace the old PFA. Th e new act will take India on the path of new regulatory framework to make it capable of global competition(5).

On the other hand in United States the Watershed legislation was passed in 1994 to regulate the manufacture and marketing of nutraceuticals. This law, known as the Dietary Supplement Health and Education Act (DSHEA), reversed 45 years of increasing FDA regulation of health-related products(6). Th e passage of the Food and Drug Administration Modernization Act of 1997 (FDAMA) made additional options available to the manufacturers of nutraceuticals. Th is legislation was the result of a reform eff ort that spanned nearly two decades. It brings about a balance in FDA regulations between approving therapeutic products so that they can benefi t patients and protecting public health by assuring that those products are safe and eff ective(7). In 1993, the Ministry of Health and Welfare in Japan established a policy of "Foods for Specifi ed Health Uses" (FOSHU) by which health claims of some selected functional foods are legally permitted. In 2001, a new regulatory system, foods with health claims (FHC) with a 'foods with nutrient function claims' (FNFC) system and newly established FOSHU was introduced. In addition, the Govt. changed the existing FOSHU, FNFC and other systems in 2005. Such changes include the new Subsystems of FOSHU such as

• Standardized FOSHU

• Qualifi ed FOSHU

• Disease risk reduction claims for FOSHU

Definitions and Categorization : Defining nutraceuticals accurately is the first step towards effective regulation. Different countries may adopt distinct definitions, leading to discrepancies in the classification of products. Some nations consider nutraceuticals as a subset of dietary supplements, while others categorize them as functional foods. Clear and universally accepted definitions can facilitate harmonization in global regulatory efforts.

Registration and Approval Requirements : The process for registering nutraceutical products varies based on the regulatory system of each country. Some countries require pre-market approval, involving rigorous safety and efficacy evaluations, while others follow a notification-based system for market entry. The choice of regulatory pathway often depends on factors such as product ingredients, health claims, and intended use.

Labeling and Health Claims : Accurate and informative labeling is crucial to ensure consumer safety and informed decision-making. Nutraceutical labels should include essential information about the product's ingredients, recommended dosage, contraindications, and potential side effects. Health claims, such as those related to disease prevention or treatment, require scientific substantiation and are subject to regulatory scrutiny.

Safety Assessments and Adverse Event Reporting : Ensuring the safety of nutraceutical products is paramount. Manufacturers are responsible for conducting safety assessments and monitoring adverse events associated with their products. Regulatory agencies play a vital role in evaluating safety data, issuing recalls if necessary, and maintaining databases of adverse events to identify potential risks.

Quality Control and Good Manufacturing Practices (GMP) : Implementing Good Manufacturing Practices is essential for ensuring the quality, consistency, and purity of nutraceutical products. Adhering to GMP guidelines helps prevent contamination, adulteration, and mislabeling, ultimately safeguarding consumer health.

Regulatory aspects of nutraceuticals or food supplements vary from country to country, and each region has its own set of rules and requirements. Here is an overview of the regulatory landscape in the United States, the Association of South East Asian Nations (ASEAN), Japan, China, Australia/New Zealand, and India:

United States

Regulatory Body: In the United States, the Food and Drug Administration (FDA) regulates nutraceuticals and dietary supplements.

Requirements

Dietary Supplement Health and Education Act (DSHEA): This act defines dietary supplements and sets forth regulations regarding their safety, labeling, and marketing claims.

Current Good Manufacturing Practices (cGMPs) : Manufa-cturers must follow cGMP regulations to ensure quality and safety in the production of dietary supplements.

Labeling Requirements : Dietary supplement labels must include a Supplement Facts panel and adhere to specific labeling guidelines provided by the FDA.

Association of South East Asian Nations (ASEAN) :

Regulatory Body: ASEAN does not have a centralized regulatory authority for nutraceuticals. Each member country has its own regulatory body responsible for regulating these products.

Requirements

ASEAN Guidelines for Traditional Medicines and Health Supplements: ASEAN countries follow these guidelines to regulate traditional medicines and health supplements, including nutraceuticals.

Each member country may have specific regulations and requirements for registration, labeling, and claims of nutraceutical products.

Japan

Regulatory Body : In Japan, nutraceuticals and food supplements fall under the category of "Foods for Specified Health Uses" (FOSHU), and they are regulated by the Consumer Affairs Agency (CAA) and the Ministry of Health, Labour, and Welfare (MHLW).

Requirements

FOSHU Approval : Manufacturers must apply for FOSHU approval, providing scientific evidence to support the health claims of the product.

Labeling Requirements : Specific labeling rules and health claims are allowed only after obtaining FOSHU approval.

China

Regulatory Body : In China, nutraceuticals and food supplements are regulated by the China Food and Drug Administration (CFDA) - now known as the National Medical Products Administration (NMPA).

Requirements

Health Food Product Approval: Manufacturers must obtain an approval certificate for health food products, which includes nutraceuticals, from the NMPA.

Health Claims : Specific health claims are allowed after obtaining the health food product approval.

Australia/New Zealand

Regulatory Body : In Australia, food supplements and nutraceuticals are regulated by Food Standards Australia New Zealand (FSANZ) and the Therapeutic Goods Administration (TGA).

Requirements

Complementary Medicines : Depending on the product's ingredients and claims, nutraceuticals may be categorized as either food or complementary medicines. Complementary medicines have stricter regulations and require TGA approval.

Listed vs. Registered Medicines : Nutraceuticals can be either listed or registered with the TGA, depending on their ingredients and health claims.

India

Regulatory Body : In India, nutraceuticals and food supplements are regulated by the Food Safety and Standards Authority of India (FSSAI).

Requirements

Nutraceutical Regulations : Nutraceuticals are categorized as Food for Special Dietary Use (FSDU) or Food for Special Medical Purpose (FSMP), and they must comply with specific regulations based on their category.

Labeling Requirements : The packaging and labeling of nutraceuticals must follow the guidelines set by the FSSAI.

It's important to note that regulations are subject to change, so manufacturers and distributors of nutraceuticals/food supplements must stay up-to-date with the latest requirements in each country or region they operate in. Consulting with regulatory experts and local authorities is crucial to ensure compliance with all applicable laws and regulations.

FSSAI Registration and Licensing for Food Supplements & Nutraceuticals - Overview

The Food Safety and Standards Authority of India (FSSAI) is the regulatory body responsible for overseeing food-related licensing in India. Any entity involved in the manufacturing, importing, distributing, or wholesaling of food supplements and nutraceuticals must obtain a valid FSSAI License.

To prevent non-compliance and ensure the safety of food products, FSSAI requires Food Business Operators (FBOs) to follow guidelines and obtain the necessary licenses. Holding an FSSAI License signifies that the food is verified and safe for consumption. It also facilitates record-keeping of licenses and compliance-related activities such as food safety audits, annual returns, product testing, and recalls. FBOs can ensure adherence to FSSAI guidelines through the licensing process, resulting in safe food consumption and informed choices for consumers while fostering fair competition among FBOs.

The application process for obtaining an FSSAI License involves the following steps:

- Submission: The applicant must fill out Form B and provide the required documents and FSSAI Licensing fees to the Food Authority.

- Unique Application Reference Number: After submission, the FBO receives a Unique Application Reference Number.

- Application Scrutiny: The Food Authority reviews the submitted application.

- Rectification: If there are any incomplete or non-compliant aspects in the application, the Licensing Authority issues a notice, allowing the FBOs 30 days to rectify and complete the application to avoid rejection.

- Inspection: Following the scrutiny, the Licensing Authority appoints a Food Safety Officer to inspect the premises and prepare an inspection report.

- License Granting: After a satisfactory inspection, the Licensing Authority grants the FSSAI License to the applicant, typically within 60 to 90 days.

- By adhering to the FSSAI regulations and obtaining the necessary licenses, FBOs contribute to the overall safety and integrity of the food supplement and nutraceutical industry in India.

List of ingredients as nutraceuticals

PART A				
S. No.	Nutraceutical ingredients	Common name	Purity Criteria	Permitted Range
1.	Astaxanthin (from *Haematococus pluvalis*), powder or oleoresin	-	Astaxanthin content	4 mg/day, Max
2.	Boswellia serrate - gum resin extract	Salai guggul / Kundru	Total boswelic acids or 11-keto-beta boswelic acids content	250 - 1,500 mg extract/day
3.	Caffiene	Caffiene	Per cent caffiene	Within levels specified in FSS Regulations
4.	Chromium picolinate/ nicotinate	-	Chromium picolinate/ nicotinate content	200 - 400 mcg / day
5.	*Cimicifuga racemosa (or Actaea racemosa). Extracted from rhizomes and roots*	*Black cohosh*	Total triterpene glycosides (minimum 0.4%), calculated as 23-epl-26-deoxyactein).	40 - 200 mg /day, Max
6.	*Citrus Bioflavonoids (Citrus x paradisi, Citrus reticulata x maxima, C. x sinensis and Citrus limon)*	Citrus	*Bioflavinoids and total polyphenol content*	150 - 600 mg / day, Max
7.	*CoQ10 from non GM source*	Co enzyme Q10	*Ubiqinone and ubiqinol content*	100-1,000 mg / day, Max
8.	Echinacea (*E. angustifolia, E. purpurea, and E. pallida*) Liquid/powder extract	Echinacea	Alkamides (0.25 mg/ml) and cichoric acid (2.5 mg/ml), if the extract used is in liquid form. In case of Hydroethanolic Echinacea extract is in a powdered form computation may be done proportionately to the weight/weight dry powder extract based on liquid	900 mg / day, Max

Table 1: Section VI of FSSAI explains some list of ingredients as nutraceuticals are as follows

References
1. ASEAN Guidelines for Traditional Medicines and Health Supplements: https://www.asean.org/storage/2017/02/6.-ASEAN-Guidelines-for-Traditional-Medicines-and-Health-Supplements.pdf
2. Australia/New Zealand (Food Standards Australia New Zealand - FSANZ and Therapeutic Goods Administration - TGA):
3. China (National Medical Products Administration - NMPA):
4. Complementary Medicines Regulation: https://www.tga.gov.au/ complementary-medicines
5. FDA's Dietary Supplements: https://www.fda.gov/food/dietary-supplements
6. India (Food Safety and Standards Authority of India - FSSAI):
7. Japan (Consumer Affairs Agency - CAA and Ministry of Health, Labour, and Welfare - MHLW):
8. Listed vs. Registered Medicines: https://www.tga.gov.au/book-page/15-listed-or-registered
9. Nutraceutical Regulations: https://www.fssai.gov.in/upload/food/Regulations/Nutraceuticals_Regulations.pdf
10. Overview of Foods for Specified Health Uses (FOSHU): https://www.caa.go.jp/en/foods/pdf/a3120914e.pdf
11. Regulations on the Registration and Management of Health Food: http://eng.sfda.gov.cn/WS03/CL0768/10588.html
12. https://cliniexperts.com/india-regulatory-services/food/food-supplements-license-fssai-registration-for-nutraceuticals-form-c/

Chapter-18

Global Market of Nutraceuticals in the Present Era

Introduction

Nutraceuticals are products that contain ingredients that have physiological benefits or provide health beyond basic nutrition. They are often consumed in the form of dietary supplements, functional foods, or beverages. The global nutraceuticals market is growing rapidly, driven by a number of factors, including:

- The increasing demand for preventive healthcare
- The rising incidence of lifestyle-related disorders
- The growing consumer focus on health-promoting diets
- Technological advancements in the production of nutraceuticals
- Regulatory support for nutraceuticals

In this chapter, we will discuss the global market of nutraceuticals in the present era. We will provide an overview of the market, including its size, share, growth, trends, and forecast. We will also discuss the key drivers and challenges of the market, as well as the competitive landscape.

Market Size and Growth

The global nutraceuticals market was valued at USD 291.33 billion in 2022 and is expected to reach USD 599.71 billion by 2030, growing at a CAGR of 9.4% during the forecast period (2023-2030). The market is segmented by product type, form, sales channel, and region.

By Product Type

The functional beverages segment is the largest segment of the global nutraceuticals market, accounting for over 30% of the market in 2022. This is due to the increasing demand for beverages that provide health benefits, such as energy, weight management, and immunity. The functional foods segment is the second largest segment, accounting for over 25% of the market in 2022. This is due to the increasing demand for foods that are naturally fortified with nutrients and provide health benefits. The dietary supplements segment is the third largest segment, accounting for over 20% of the market in 2022. This is due to the increasing demand for products that provide specific nutrients or other health-promoting compounds.

By Form

The capsules and tablets segment is the largest segment of the global nutraceuticals market, accounting for over 40% of the market in 2022. This is due to the convenience and portability of capsules and tablets. The liquid segment is the second largest segment, accounting for over 25% of the market in 2022. This is due to the increasing demand for liquid nutraceuticals, such as sports drinks and energy drinks. The powder segment is the third largest segment, accounting for over 20% of the market in 2022. This is due to the increasing demand for powders that can be added to foods or beverages.

By Sales Channel

The hypermarkets and supermarkets segment is the largest segment of the global nutraceuticals market, accounting for over 40% of the market in 2022. This is due to the wide availability of nutraceuticals in hypermarkets and supermarkets. The specialty stores segment is the second largest segment, accounting for over 25% of the market in 2022. This is due to the increasing number of specialty stores that sell nutraceuticals. The pharmacies segment is the third largest segment, accounting for over 20% of the market in 2022. This is due to the fact that pharmacies are a trusted source of health information and products.

By Region

North America is the largest market for nutraceuticals, accounting for over 35% of the market in 2022. This is due to the high awareness of the benefits of nutraceuticals and the availability of a wide range of products in the region. Europe is the second largest market for nutraceuticals, accounting for over 25% of the market in 2022. This is due to the increasing awareness of the benefits of nutraceuticals and the growing demand for preventive healthcare in the region. Asia-Pacific is the third largest market for nutraceuticals, accounting for over 20% of the market in 2022. This is due to the growing middle class and the increasing demand for health-promoting products in the region. Latin America and Middle East & Africa are the smaller markets for nutraceuticals, but they are expected to grow at a faster pace than the other regions in the coming years.

Statistics data on nutraceuticals production in different countries :

Country	Production Value (USD)	Growth Rate (CAGR)
China	114.3 billion	10%
United States	85.9 billion	9%
Japan	42.7 billion	8%
Germany	37.5 billion	7%
France	32.6 billion	6%
Brazil	27.1 billion	5%
India	22.9 billion	4%
Canada	17.8 billion	3%
South Korea	16.2 billion	2%

These statistics are for the year 2022. It is important to note that the nutraceuticals market is constantly evolving, so these statistics may change from year to year.

Key Drivers of Nutraceuticals Production

The following are some of the key drivers of nutraceuticals production :

• **Increasing demand for preventive healthcare** : Consumers are becoming more aware of the importance of preventive healthcare and are looking for ways to improve their overall health and well-being. Nutraceuticals can play a role in preventive healthcare by providing essential nutrients and other health-promoting compounds.

• **Rising incidence of lifestyle-related disorders** : The incidence of lifestyle-related disorders, such as obesity, heart disease, and diabetes, is increasing in many parts of the world. Nutraceuticals can be used to manage these conditions and improve overall health.

• **Growing consumer focus on health-promoting diets**: Consumers are becoming more interested in eating healthy diets that include nutraceuticals. This is due to the increasing awareness of the benefits of nutraceuticals and the growing availability of these products.

• **Technological advancements in nutraceuticals production** : Technological advancements have made it possible to produce nutraceuticals that are more effective and affordable. This has led to an increase in nutraceuticals production.

• **Regulatory support for nutraceuticals** : In many countries, there is increasing regulatory support for nutraceuticals. This has created a more favorable environment for nutraceuticals production.

Graphical representation of nutraceuticals consumption in different areas of the world :

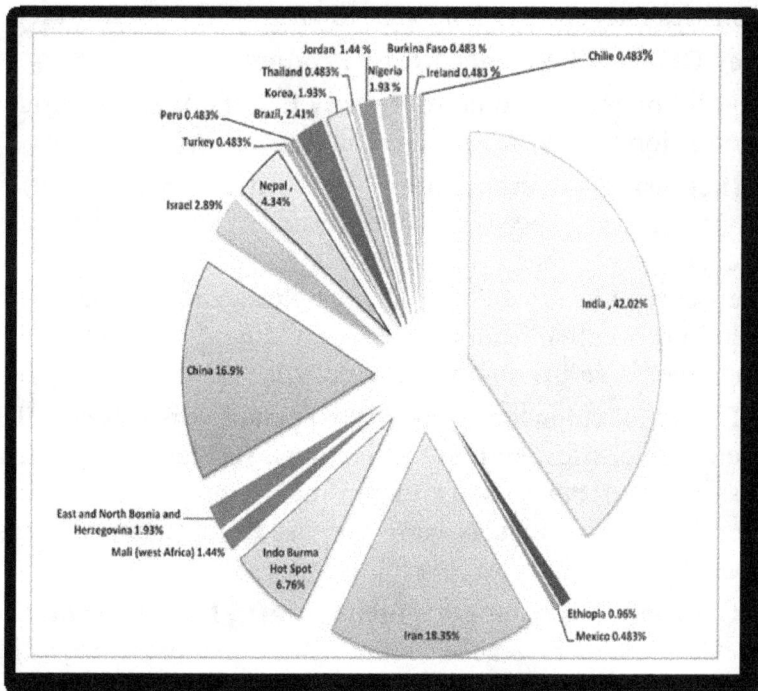

The pie chart shows that Asia-Pacific is the largest market for nutraceuticals, accounting for 32.4% of global consumption in 2022. This is followed by North America (29.7%), Europe (23.7%), Latin America (9.8%), and Middle East & Africa (4.4%).

The high consumption of nutraceuticals in Asia-Pacific is due to the region's large and growing population, as well as the increasing awareness of the benefits of nutraceuticals. North America and Europe also have a high consumption of nutraceuticals, due to the region's high standards of living and the increasing demand for preventive healthcare.

Latin America and Middle East & Africa have a lower consumption of nutraceuticals, but these regions are expected to grow at a faster pace in the coming years. This is

252

due to the increasing awareness of the benefits of nutraceuticals and the growing middle class in these regions.

Here are some additional details about the nutraceuticals consumption in different areas of the world:

• **Asia-Pacific** : The high consumption of nutraceuticals in Asia-Pacific is driven by a number of factors, including the region's large and growing population, the increasing awareness of the benefits of nutraceuticals, and the growing demand for preventive healthcare. The top nutraceuticals consumed in Asia-Pacific are vitamins, minerals, and dietary supplements.

• **North America** : The consumption of nutraceuticals in North America is also high. The top nutraceuticals consumed in North America are vitamins, minerals, and dietary supplements. The high consumption of nutraceuticals in North America is driven by the region's high standards of living, the increasing demand for preventive healthcare, and the large and growing population.

• **Europe** : The consumption of nutraceuticals in Europe is also high. The top nutraceuticals consumed in Europe are vitamins, minerals, and dietary supplements. The high consumption of nutraceuticals in Europe is driven by the region's high standards of living, the increasing demand for preventive healthcare, and the large and growing population.

• **Latin America** : The consumption of nutraceuticals in Latin America is lower than in other regions, but it is expected to grow at a faster pace in the coming years. The top nutraceuticals consumed in Latin America are vitamins, minerals, and dietary supplements. The growth of the nutraceuticals market in Latin America is being driven by the increasing awareness of the benefits of nutraceuticals, the growing middle class, and the increasing demand for preventive healthcare.

• **Middle East & Africa :** The consumption of nutraceuticals in Middle East & Africa is the lowest among all regions. However, the market is expected to grow at a faster pace in the coming years. The top nutraceuticals consumed in Middle East & Africa are vitamins, minerals, and dietary supplements. The growth of the nutraceuticals market in Middle East & Africa is being driven by the increasing awareness of the benefits of nutraceuticals, the growing middle class, and the increasing demand for preventive healthcare.

Nutraceutical scenario in India

Th e Indian nutraceutical industry has great prospects. Over the last decade a wide range of products have been available, giving an insight into the tremendous growth. On one hand a booming economy has resulted in overall increase in disposable income of population. Added to this unhealthy, eating habits coupled with sedentary lifestyle have led to increase incidence of diet and its related health issues. On the other hand, there is a growing awareness on the importance of nutrition and diet for long term good health. Th ese have contributed to a favorable market conditions for Nutraceutical industry in India. India has a lot of advantages like qualified human resources, world class R & D facilities and varied raw material-aspects that give our country a leading edge. Th e Indian Nutritional market is estimated to be USD 1 Billion. While the global market is growing at a CAGR of 7%, the Indian market has been growing much faster at a CAGR of 18% for the last three years, driven by Functional food and beverages categories. However the latent market in India is two to four times the current market size and is between USD 2 to USD 4 billion with almost 148 million potential customers. In USD 1 billion market size functional food having 54% market share followed by 32% market share of Dietary supplement and 14% share of Functional beverages. Th e Indian nutraceutical market is dominated primarily by pharmaceuticals and FMCG companies with very few pure play nutraceutical companies. Some major companies Marketing Nutraceuticals in India are GlaxoSmithKline consumer healthcare, Dabur India, Cadila Health care, EID Parry's, Zandu Pharmaceuticals, Himalaya herbal Healthcare, Amway, Sami labs, Elder pharmaceuticals and Ranbaxy

Some famous nutraceuticals production companies, their products, and their income :

Company	Products	Revenue (inUSD) (2022)
Amway	Nutrilite, BodyKey, Artistry	8.4 billion
Herbalife	Herbalife Nutrition, Herbalife24	5.4 billion
GNC	Vitamin World, Total Gym	4.1 billion
Abbott Laboratories	Ensure, Similac, Glucerna	3.9 billion
Pfizer	Centrum, Robitussin, Lipitor	3.8 billion
Nature's Bounty	Centrum, Alive!, Osteo Bi-Flex	3.6 billion
Unilever	Dove, Axe, Hellmann's	2.9 billion
Nestlé	Nespresso, Nescafé, KitKat	2.8 billion
Bayer	Aleve, Claritin, Bayer Back & Body	2.6 billion

These companies produce a wide range of nutraceutical products, including vitamins, minerals, dietary supplements, functional foods, and beverages. Their products are available in a variety of forms, such as capsules, tablets, powders, liquids, and gummies.

The revenue of these companies varies depending on their product portfolio, geographic reach, and marketing strategies. However, all of these companies are major players in the global nutraceuticals market.

Here are some additional details about these companies:

- Amway: Amway is a direct-selling company that sells a wide range of products, including nutraceuticals. The company's flagship nutraceutical brand is Nutrilite, which sells vitamins, minerals, and dietary supplements. Amway's revenue in 2022 was 8.4 billion USD.

- Herbalife: Herbalife is another direct-selling company that sells nutraceuticals. The company's flagship nutraceutical brand is Herbalife Nutrition, which sells weight management products, sports nutrition products, and nutritional supplements. Herbalife's revenue in 2022 was 5.4 billion USD.

- GNC: GNC is a retail store that sells a wide range of nutraceuticals, including vitamins, minerals, dietary supplements, and sports nutrition products. The company also has a private label brand called BodyTech. GNC's revenue in 2022 was 4.1 billion USD.

- Abbott Laboratories: Abbott Laboratories is a pharmaceutical company that sells a wide range of medical products, including nutraceuticals. The company's flagship nutraceutical brand is Ensure, which sells nutritional shakes and drinks for people with special dietary needs. Abbott Laboratories' revenue in 2022 was 3.9 billion USD.

- Pfizer: Pfizer is a pharmaceutical company that sells a wide range of prescription and over-the-counter medications, including nutraceuticals. The company's flagship nutraceutical brand is Centrum, which sells multivitamins and minerals. Pfizer's revenue in 2022 was 3.8 billion USD.

Challenges to Nutraceuticals Production

The following are some of the challenges to nutraceuticals production:

• **Lack of awareness about nutraceuticals :** There is still a lack of awareness about nutraceuticals among consumers in many parts of the world. This can be a barrier to the growth of the nutraceuticals market.

• **High cost of some nutraceuticals :** Some nutraceuticals can be expensive, which can make them inaccessible to some consumers.

• **Regulatory challenges :** There are still some regulatory challenges to nutraceuticals production in some countries. This can make it difficult for companies to market and sell nutraceuticals in these countries.

Despite these challenges, the nutraceuticals market is expected to continue to grow in the coming years. The growth of the market will be driven by the factors mentioned above.

Conclusion

The global nutraceuticals market is growing rapidly, driven by a number of factors, including the increasing demand for preventive healthcare, the rising incidence of lifestyle-related disorders, the growing consumer focus on health-promoting diets, and technological advancements in the production of nutraceuticals.

The market is segmented by product type, form, sales channel, and region. Functional beverages, functional foods, and dietary supplements are the three main product segments. Capsules and tablets, liquid, powder, and others are the four primary form segments. Hypermarkets and supermarkets, specialty stores, pharmacies, and online channels are the four main sales channel segments. Asia-Pacific, North America, Europe, Latin America, and the Middle East and Africa are the five main regional segments.

The market is facing a number of challenges, such as the lack of awareness of nutraceuticals among consumers, the high cost of some nutraceuticals, and regulatory challenges. However, the market is expected to continue to grow in the coming years due to the factors mentioned above.

Here are some of the key trends that are expected to shape the global nutraceuticals market in the coming years:

• **The increasing demand for personalized nutraceuticals** : Consumers are becoming more interested in personalized nutraceuticals that are tailored to their individual needs and health goals. This trend is being driven by the growing availability of genetic testing and other technologies that can help personalize nutraceuticals.

• **The growing demand for vegan and vegetarian nutraceuticals** : The number of vegans and vegetarians is growing rapidly, and this is driving the demand for vegan and vegetarian nutraceuticals. These products are made without animal products, and they are becoming increasingly available in mainstream retail stores.

• **The increasing demand for nutraceuticals for specific health conditions** : Consumers are becoming more aware of the potential benefits of nutraceuticals for specific health conditions, such as heart disease, diabetes, and cancer. This is driving the demand for nutraceuticals that are specifically designed to address these conditions.

• **The increasing demand for nutraceuticals for sports performance** : Athletes and fitness enthusiasts are increasingly using nutraceuticals to improve their performance. These products can provide energy, boost endurance, and reduce muscle soreness.

The global nutraceuticals market is a dynamic and growing market. The trends mentioned above are expected to shape the market in the coming years.

References

1. FICCI-Ernst & Young study: Nutraceuticals-Critical supplement for building a healthy India, Health Foods and Dietary Supplements Association conferences, Mumbai Sep10, 2009.
2. Global Nutraceuticals Market Size, Share, Growth, Trends, and Forecast-2022-203: https://www.thebusinessresearchcompany.com/report/nutraceuticals-global-market-report
3. Nutraceuticals Market - Global Industry Analysis, Size, Share, Growth, Trends, and Forecast 2022-2030: https://www.alliedmarketresearch.com/nutraceuticals-market
4. Nutraceuticals Market - Growth, Trends, COVID-19 Impact, and Forecasts (2022-2028): https://www.marketresearch.com/Food-Beverage-c84/Food-c167/Nutraceuticals-c503/
5. Nutraceuticals Market Size, Share & Trends | Report, 2022-2030: https://www.thebusinessresearchcompany.com/report/nutraceuticals-global-market-report

www.ingramcontent.com/pod-product-compliance
Lightning Source LLC
Chambersburg PA
CBHW050213270326
41914CB00003BA/396